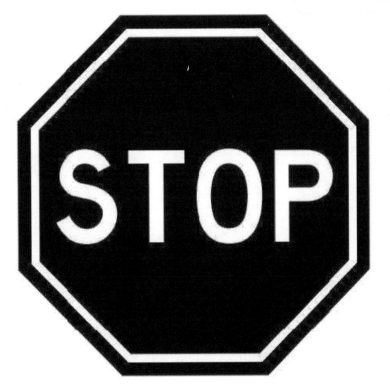

FREE Test Taking Tips DVD Offer

To help us better serve you, we have developed a Test Taking Tips DVD that we would like to give you for FREE. **This DVD covers world-class test taking tips that you can use to be even more successful when you are taking your test.**

All that we ask is that you email us your feedback about your study guide. Please let us know what you thought about it – whether that is good, bad or indifferent.

To get your **FREE Test Taking Tips DVD**, email freedvd@studyguideteam.com with "FREE DVD" in the subject line and the following information in the body of the email:

> a. The title of your study guide.
>
> b. Your product rating on a scale of 1-5, with 5 being the highest rating.
>
> c. Your feedback about the study guide. What did you think of it?
>
> d. Your full name and shipping address to send your free DVD.

If you have any questions or concerns, please don't hesitate to contact us at freedvd@studyguideteam.com.

Thanks again!

MCAT CARS Review
Study Guide

MCAT Critical Analysis & Reasoning Skills (Verbal) Team

Table of Contents

Quick Overview

As you draw closer to taking your exam, effective preparation becomes more and more important. Thankfully, you have this study guide to help you get ready. Use this guide to help keep your studying on track and refer to it often.

This study guide contains several key sections that will help you be successful on your exam. The guide contains tips for what you should do the night before and the day of the test. Also included are test-taking tips. Knowing the right information is not always enough. Many well-prepared test takers struggle with exams. These tips will help equip you to accurately read, assess, and answer test questions.

A large part of the guide is devoted to showing you what content to expect on the exam and to helping you better understand that content. Near the end of this guide is a practice test so that you can see how well you have grasped the content. Then, answer explanations are provided so that you can understand why you missed certain questions.

Don't try to cram the night before you take your exam. This is not a wise strategy for a few reasons. First, your retention of the information will be low. Your time would be better used by reviewing information you already know rather than trying to learn a lot of new information. Second, you will likely become stressed as you try to gain a large amount of knowledge in a short amount of time. Third, you will be depriving yourself of sleep. So be sure to go to bed at a reasonable time the night before. Being well-rested helps you focus and remain calm.

Be sure to eat a substantial breakfast the morning of the exam. If you are taking the exam in the afternoon, be sure to have a good lunch as well. Being hungry is distracting and can make it difficult to focus. You have hopefully spent lots of time preparing for the exam. Don't let an empty stomach get in the way of success!

When travelling to the testing center, leave earlier than needed. That way, you have a buffer in case you experience any delays. This will help you remain calm and will keep you from missing your appointment time at the testing center.

Be sure to pace yourself during the exam. Don't try to rush through the exam. There is no need to risk performing poorly on the exam just so you can leave the testing center early. Allow yourself to use all of the allotted time if needed.

Remain positive while taking the exam even if you feel like you are performing poorly. Thinking about the content you should have mastered will not help you perform better on the exam.

Once the exam is complete, take some time to relax. Even if you feel that you need to take the exam again, you will be well served by some down time before you begin studying again. It's often easier to convince yourself to study if you know that it will come with a reward!

Test-Taking Strategies

1. Predicting the Answer

When you feel confident in your preparation for a multiple-choice test, try predicting the answer before reading the answer choices. This is especially useful on questions that test objective factual knowledge or that ask you to fill in a blank. By predicting the answer before reading the available choices, you eliminate the possibility that you will be distracted or led astray by an incorrect answer choice. You will feel more confident in your selection if you read the question, predict the answer, and then find your prediction among the answer choices. After using this strategy, be sure to still read all of the answer choices carefully and completely. If you feel unprepared, you should not attempt to predict the answers. This would be a waste of time and an opportunity for your mind to wander in the wrong direction.

2. Reading the Whole Question

Too often, test takers scan a multiple-choice question, recognize a few familiar words, and immediately jump to the answer choices. Test authors are aware of this common impatience, and they will sometimes prey upon it. For instance, a test author might subtly turn the question into a negative, or he or she might redirect the focus of the question right at the end. The only way to avoid falling into these traps is to read the entirety of the question carefully before reading the answer choices.

3. Looking for Wrong Answers

Long and complicated multiple-choice questions can be intimidating. One way to simplify a difficult multiple-choice question is to eliminate all of the answer choices that are clearly wrong. In most sets of answers, there will be at least one selection that can be dismissed right away. If the test is administered on paper, the test taker could draw a line through it to indicate that it may be ignored; otherwise, the test taker will have to perform this operation mentally or on scratch paper. In either case, once the obviously incorrect answers have been eliminated, the remaining choices may be considered. Sometimes identifying the clearly wrong answers will give the test taker some information about the correct answer. For instance, if one of the remaining answer choices is a direct opposite of one of the eliminated answer choices, it may well be the correct answer. The opposite of obviously wrong is obviously right! Of course, this is not always the case. Some answers are obviously incorrect simply because they are irrelevant to the question being asked. Still, identifying and eliminating some incorrect answer choices is a good way to simplify a multiple-choice question.

4. Don't Overanalyze

Anxious test takers often overanalyze questions. When you are nervous, your brain will often run wild, causing you to make associations and discover clues that don't actually exist. If you feel that this may be a problem for you, do whatever you can to slow down during the test. Try taking a deep breath or counting to ten. As you read and consider the question, restrict yourself to the particular words used by the author. Avoid thought tangents about what the author *really* meant, or what he or she was *trying* to say. The only things that matter on a multiple-choice test are the words that are actually in the question. You must avoid reading too much into a multiple-choice question, or supposing that the writer meant something other than what he or she wrote.

5. No Need for Panic

It is wise to learn as many strategies as possible before taking a multiple-choice test, but it is likely that you will come across a few questions for which you simply don't know the answer. In this situation, avoid panicking. Because most multiple-choice tests include dozens of questions, the relative value of a single wrong answer is small. Moreover, your failure on one question has no effect on your success elsewhere on the test. As much as possible, you should compartmentalize each question on a multiple-choice test. In other words, you should not allow your feelings about one question to affect your success on the others. When you find a question that you either don't understand or don't know how to answer, just take a deep breath and do your best. Read the entire question slowly and carefully. Try rephrasing the question a couple of different ways. Then, read all of the answer choices carefully. After eliminating obviously wrong answers, make a selection and move on to the next question.

6. Confusing Answer Choices

When working on a difficult multiple-choice question, there may be a tendency to focus on the answer choices that are the easiest to understand. Many people, whether consciously or not, gravitate to the answer choices that require the least concentration, knowledge, and memory. This is a mistake. When you come across an answer choice that is confusing, you should give it extra attention. A question might be confusing because you do not know the subject matter to which it refers. If this is the case, don't eliminate the answer before you have affirmatively settled on another. When you come across an answer choice of this type, set it aside as you look at the remaining choices. If you can confidently assert that one of the other choices is correct, you can leave the confusing answer aside. Otherwise, you will need to take a moment to try to better understand the confusing answer choice. Rephrasing is one way to tease out the sense of a confusing answer choice.

7. Your First Instinct

Many people struggle with multiple-choice tests because they overthink the questions. If you have studied sufficiently for the test, you should be prepared to trust your first instinct once you have carefully and completely read the question and all of the answer choices. There is a great deal of research suggesting that the mind can come to the correct conclusion very quickly once it has obtained all of the relevant information. At times, it may seem to you as if your intuition is working faster even than your reasoning mind. This may in fact be true. The knowledge you obtain while studying may be retrieved from your subconscious before you have a chance to work out the associations that support it. Verify your instinct by working out the reasons that it should be trusted.

8. Key Words

Many test takers struggle with multiple-choice questions because they have poor reading comprehension skills. Quickly reading and understanding a multiple-choice question requires a mixture of skill and experience. To help with this, try jotting down a few key words and phrases on a piece of scrap paper. Doing this concentrates the process of reading and forces the mind to weigh the relative importance of the question's parts. In selecting words and phrases to write down, the test taker thinks about the question more deeply and carefully. This is especially true for multiple-choice questions that are preceded by a long prompt.

9. Subtle Negatives

One of the oldest tricks in the multiple-choice test writer's book is to subtly reverse the meaning of a question with a word like *not* or *except*. If you are not paying attention to each word in the question, you can easily be led astray by this trick. For instance, a common question format is, "Which of the following is...?" Obviously, if the question instead is, "Which of the following is not...?," then the answer will be quite different. Even worse, the test makers are aware of the potential for this mistake and will include one answer choice that would be correct if the question were not negated or reversed. A test taker who misses the reversal will find what he or she believes to be a correct answer and will be so confident that he or she will fail to reread the question and discover the original error. The only way to avoid this is to practice a wide variety of multiple-choice questions and to pay close attention to each and every word.

10. Reading Every Answer Choice

It may seem obvious, but you should always read every one of the answer choices! Too many test takers fall into the habit of scanning the question and assuming that they understand the question because they recognize a few key words. From there, they pick the first answer choice that answers the question they believe they have read. Test takers who read all of the answer choices might discover that one of the latter answer choices is actually *more* correct. Moreover, reading all of the answer choices can remind you of facts related to the question that can help you arrive at the correct answer. Sometimes, a misstatement or incorrect detail in one of the latter answer choices will trigger your memory of the subject and will enable you to find the right answer. Failing to read all of the answer choices is like not reading all of the items on a restaurant menu: you might miss out on the perfect choice.

11. Spot the Hedges

One of the keys to success on multiple-choice tests is paying close attention to every word. This is never more true than with words like *almost*, *most*, *some*, and *sometimes*. These words are called "hedges" because they indicate that a statement is not totally true or not true in every place and time. An absolute statement will contain no hedges, but in many subjects, like literature and history, the answers are not always straightforward or absolute. There are always exceptions to the rules in these subjects. For this reason, you should favor those multiple-choice questions that contain hedging language. The presence of qualifying words indicates that the author is taking special care with his or her words, which is certainly important when composing the right answer. After all, there are many ways to be wrong, but there is only one way to be right! For this reason, it is wise to avoid answers that are absolute when taking a multiple-choice test. An absolute answer is one that says things are either all one way or all another. They often include words like *every*, *always*, *best*, and *never*. If you are taking a multiple-choice test in a subject that doesn't lend itself to absolute answers, be on your guard if you see any of these words.

12. Long Answers

In many subject areas, the answers are not simple. As already mentioned, the right answer often requires hedges. Another common feature of the answers to a complex or subjective question are qualifying clauses, which are groups of words that subtly modify the meaning of the sentence. If the question or answer choice describes a rule to which there are exceptions or the subject matter is complicated, ambiguous, or confusing, the correct answer will require many words in order to be expressed clearly and accurately. In essence, you should not be deterred by answer choices that seem excessively long. Oftentimes, the author of the text will not be able to write the correct answer without offering some qualifications and modifications. Your job is to read the answer choices thoroughly and completely and to select the one that most accurately and precisely answers the question.

13. Restating to Understand

Sometimes, a question on a multiple-choice test is difficult not because of what it asks but because of how it is written. If this is the case, restate the question or answer choice in different words. This process serves a couple of important purposes. First, it forces you to concentrate on the core of the question. In order to rephrase the question accurately, you have to understand it well. Rephrasing the question will concentrate your mind on the key words and ideas. Second, it will present the information to your mind in a fresh way. This process may trigger your memory and render some useful scrap of information picked up while studying.

14. True Statements

Sometimes an answer choice will be true in itself, but it does not answer the question. This is one of the main reasons why it is essential to read the question carefully and completely before proceeding to the answer choices. Too often, test takers skip ahead to the answer choices and look for true statements. Having found one of these, they are content to select it without reference to the question above. Obviously, this provides an easy way for test makers to play tricks. The savvy test taker will always read the entire question before turning to the answer choices. Then, having settled on a correct answer choice, he or she will refer to the original question and ensure that the selected answer is relevant. The mistake of choosing a correct-but-irrelevant answer choice is especially common on questions related to specific pieces of objective knowledge, like historical or scientific facts. A prepared test taker will have a wealth of factual knowledge at his or her disposal, and should not be careless in its application.

15. No Patterns

One of the more dangerous ideas that circulates about multiple-choice tests is that the correct answers tend to fall into patterns. These erroneous ideas range from a belief that B and C are the most common right answers, to the idea that an unprepared test-taker should answer "A-B-A-C-A-D-A-B-A." It cannot be emphasized enough that pattern-seeking of this type is exactly the WRONG way to approach a multiple-choice test. To begin with, it is highly unlikely that the test maker will plot the correct answers according to some predetermined pattern. The questions are scrambled and delivered in a random order. Furthermore, even if the test maker was following a pattern in the assignation of correct answers, there is no reason why the test taker would know which pattern he or she was using. Any attempt to discern a pattern in the answer choices is a waste of time and a distraction from the real work of taking the test. A test taker would be much better served by extra preparation before the test than by reliance on a pattern in the answers.

FREE DVD OFFER

Don't forget that doing well on your exam includes both understanding the test content and understanding how to use what you know to do well on the test. We offer a completely FREE Test Taking Tips DVD that covers world class test taking tips that you can use to be even more successful when you are taking your test.

All that we ask is that you email us your feedback about your study guide. To get your **FREE Test Taking Tips DVD**, email freedvd@studyguideteam.com with "FREE DVD" in the subject line and the following information in the body of the email:

- The title of your study guide.
- Your product rating on a scale of 1-5, with 5 being the highest rating.
- Your feedback about the study guide. What did you think of it?
- Your full name and shipping address to send your free DVD.

The Critical Analysis and Reasoning Skills section of the MCAT provides a passage to read and asks test takers to answer questions relating to the passage after they've read it. There are 53 questions in this section and all are passage-based, following complex passages that are roughly 500-600 words in length. The purpose of the Critical Analysis and Reasoning Skills section is to test a student's ability to retain complex text information with the ability to analyze and/or synthesize it, given a certain set of questions. The questions assess *Foundations of Comprehension, Reasoning Within the Text,* and *Reasoning Beyond the Text*. Medical students and physicians are constantly confronted with difficult texts that require tedious analysis, so this section is important for test takers to learn.

The passages and questions encountered on the MCAT will be drawn roughly equally from the social sciences and humanities. While the excepts used may be taken from a variety of books and journals, the social sciences passages are typically more objective and factual, while humanities passages may be more opinionated or conversational, with a focus on relationships of ideas and changes over time. The disciplines from which the content pulls include the arts, various global cultures, ethics, philosophy, literature, religion, architecture, and popular culture, among others. While not an exhaustive list, social sciences passages are typically drawn from education, anthropology, sociology, psychology, public health, linguistics, economics, geography, history, political science, and archeology. The sections below are a comprehensive list of characteristics you will encounter in the passages. Some of the sections, such as *Main Idea* or *Words Used in Context*, should be familiar to you. However, other sections, such as *Principles that Function in the Selection* or *The Impact of New Information*, are subjects that may be unfamiliar to new MCAT test takers.

It's important to remember that it is not necessary to have outside knowledge of the passage information before entering the test. Every question relies on the universe of the passage; therefore, it's important to read the whole passage first and at least designate what the primary purpose or main idea of the passage is. If test takers delve straight into the questions, they may not have a sense of the passage's entirety, and thus will waste time reading answers that have no meaning to them.

Introduction to the MCAT

Function of the Test

All medical schools in the United States, as well as many Canadian schools, require candidates to submit Medical College Admission Test (MCAT) scores as part of the admissions process. Most schools require that an applicant's scores were obtained within the prior three years. The MCAT is a standardized test that assesses several different areas such as critical thinking and problem solving; knowledge of natural, behavioral, and social science concepts; and other principles related to the medical field. The AAMC develops and writes the MCAT. Candidate are eligible to take the MCAT if they are applying to a professional school of medicine in the following areas: allopathic, osteopathic, podiatric, or veterinary medicine. Candidates should apply and take the MCAT about a year before entering medical school. Although there are no prerequisites required to take the MCAT, the exam covers topics on introductory biology, general and organic chemistry, physics, and first-semester psychology, sociology and biochemistry; college-level science labs and statistics concepts and skills are also assessed on the MCAT.

Test Administration

The MCAT is given at hundreds of testing sites throughout the country at multiple times throughout the year between January and September. Registration for the following year typically starts in the fall prior to the year of administration. International students may apply for the MCAT if they hold a MBBS degree or are in a program to obtain an MBBS. Since the MCAT is for candidates wishing to apply to a professional medical school, there are "special permissions" granted to individuals who are not planning on attending such a school. These special requests can be granted via email to mcat@aamc.org and will typically be reviewed within five business days. Details for special requests can be viewed on the official MCAT website: https://students-residents.aamc.org/applying-medical-school/faq/mcat-faqs/

Candidates should attempt to take the exam early in the year, in case a retest is necessary. This gives a student sufficient time to study and find a second available seat. The MCAT can be taken three times in a year and four times in two consecutive years. The MCAT can be taken up to seven times in a lifetime. No shows and voids count as attempts against the candidate's test limits.

Test Format

The MCAT is a standardized, multiple-choice test. There are 230 questions and the test takes about 6 hours and 15 minutes to complete, with additional time for breaks. There are four sections on the MCAT: biological and biochemical foundations of living systems; chemical and physical foundations of biological systems; psychological, social, and biological foundations of behavior; and critical analysis and reasoning. The first three sections include scientific inquiry and reasoning skills. The following table displays the categories, number of questions, and allotted time:

Category	Number of questions	Time limit (min)
Biological and Biochemical Foundations of Living Systems	59	95
Chemical and Physical Foundations of Biological Systems	59	95
Psychological, Social, and Biological Foundations of Behavior	59	95
Critical Analysis and Reasoning Skills	53	90

Scoring

Scores for the MCAT are released approximately a month after the date the exam was taken. If the MCAT was taken in April or May, the scores take longer to reach the candidate, but a percentile ranking will be sent about three weeks after taking the exam. This will help a candidate decide if a retest is necessary. There are five scores for the MCAT exam: a score will be given for each of the four sections and one combined score will be given for the total test. The four individual sections range from 118-132 and the total score ranges from 472-528. Scores are scaled and are not curved. However, since some forms of the test are more difficult than others, raw scores are converted to scaled score, which consider test difficulty.

Recent/Future Developments

The current version of the MCAT discussed above is reflective of the latest updates from April of 2015. Periodic updates are necessary because the field of medicine continues to change and the MCAT needs to reflect these changes. The required knowledge, skills, and training that a new physician needs has changed since the MCAT's previous 1991 version, and will likely dictate future revisions.

Foundations of Comprehension

Basic Components of the Text

Main Idea or Primary Purpose

On the MCAT, some questions may ask test takers to identify the *main idea* or *primary purpose* of the passage. The main idea is what the writer wants to say about that topic. A writer may make the point that global warming is a growing problem that must be addressed in order to save the planet. Therefore, the topic is global warming, and the main idea is that *it's a serious problem needing to be addressed*. The topic can be expressed in a word or two, but the main idea should be a complete thought.

In order to illustrate the main idea, a writer will use supporting details—the details that provide evidence or examples to help make a point. Supporting details are typically found in nonfiction texts that seek to inform or persuade the reader.

For example, in the example of global warming, the author's main idea is to show the seriousness of this growing problem and the need for change. The use of supporting details in this piece would be critical in effectively making that point. Supporting details used here might include statistics on an increase in global temperatures and studies showing the impact of global warming on the planet. The author could also include projections for future climate change to illustrate potential lasting effects of global warming.

Some questions may also ask test takers to select the best title for the passage. Going back to the *topic*, for these questions it's important that test takers give a narrower answer that still encompasses the main idea of the passage. Asking for the appropriate title for passages is rare, but it's best to be prepared for anything.

Finally, the MCAT may ask test takers to summarize the passage they've read. Giving a summary is different than pointing out the main idea; in a summary, test takers should expect to choose a more comprehensive answer on the passage, one that includes the most important points. In the example of global warming, the summary might be the main idea merged with the most important supporting details. Reading the passage in its entirety before approaching the questions is key to getting a comprehensive look at what the most important aspects of the text will be.

Understanding the Development of Themes

Identifying Theme or Central Message

The *theme* is the central message of a fictional work, whether that work is structured as prose, drama, or poetry. It is the heart of what an author is trying to say to readers through the writing, and theme is largely conveyed through literary elements and techniques.

In literature, a theme can often be determined by considering the over-arching narrative conflict within the work. Though there are several types of conflicts and several potential themes within them, the following are the most common:

- *Individual against the self*—relevant to themes of self-awareness, internal struggles, pride, coming of age, facing reality, fate, free will, vanity, loss of innocence, loneliness, isolation, fulfillment, failure, and disillusionment

- *Individual against nature*— relevant to themes of knowledge vs. ignorance, nature as beauty, quest for discovery, self-preservation, chaos and order, circle of life, death, and destruction of beauty

- *Individual against society*— relevant to themes of power, beauty, good, evil, war, class struggle, totalitarianism, role of men/women, wealth, corruption, change vs. tradition, capitalism, destruction, heroism, injustice, and racism

- *Individual against another individual*— relevant to themes of hope, loss of love or hope, sacrifice, power, revenge, betrayal, and honor

For example, in Hawthorne's *The Scarlet Letter*, one possible narrative conflict could be the individual against the self, with a relevant theme of internal struggles. This theme is alluded to through characterization—Dimmesdale's moral struggle with his love for Hester and Hester's internal struggles with the truth and her daughter, Pearl. It's also alluded to through plot—Dimmesdale's suicide and Hester helping the very townspeople who initially condemned her.

Sometimes, a text can convey a *message* or *universal lesson*—a truth or insight that the reader infers from the text, based on analysis of the literary and/or poetic elements. This message is often presented as a statement. For example, a potential message in Shakespeare's *Hamlet* could be "Revenge is what ultimately drives the human soul." This message can be immediately determined through plot and characterization in numerous ways, but it can also be determined through the setting of Norway, which is bordering on war.

How Authors Develop Theme

Authors employ a variety of techniques to present a theme. They may compare or contrast characters, events, places, ideas, or historical or invented settings to speak thematically. They may use analogies, metaphors, similes, allusions, or other literary devices to convey the theme. An author's use of diction, syntax, and tone can also help convey the theme. Authors will often develop themes through the development of characters, use of the setting, repetition of ideas, use of symbols, and through contrasting value systems. Authors of both fiction and nonfiction genres will use a variety of these techniques to develop one or more themes.

Regardless of the literary genre, there are commonalities in how authors, playwrights, and poets develop themes or central ideas.

Authors often do research, the results of which contributes to theme. In prose fiction and drama, this research may include real historical information about the setting the author has chosen or include elements that make fictional characters, settings, and plots seem realistic to the reader. In nonfiction, research is critical since the information contained within this literature must be accurate and, moreover, accurately represented.

In fiction, authors present a narrative conflict that will contribute to the overall theme. In fiction, this conflict may involve the storyline itself and some trouble within characters that needs resolution. In nonfiction, this conflict may be an explanation or commentary on factual people and events.

Authors will sometimes use character motivation to convey theme, such as in the example from *Hamlet* regarding revenge. In fiction, the characters an author creates will think, speak, and act in ways that effectively convey the theme to readers. In nonfiction, the characters are factual, as in a biography, but authors pay particular attention to presenting those motivations to make them clear to readers.

Authors also use literary devices as a means of conveying theme. For example, the use of moon symbolism in Shelley's *Frankenstein* is significant as its phases can be compared to the phases that the Creature undergoes as he struggles with his identity.

The selected point of view can also contribute to a work's theme. The use of first person point of view in a fiction or non-fiction work engages the reader's response differently than third person point of view. The central idea or theme from a first-person narrative may differ from a third-person limited text.

In literary nonfiction, authors usually identify the purpose of their writing, which differs from fiction, where the general purpose is to entertain. The purpose of nonfiction is usually to inform, persuade, or entertain the audience. The stated purpose of a non-fiction text will drive how the central message or theme, if applicable, is presented.

Authors identify an audience for their writing, which is critical in shaping the theme of the work. For example, the audience for J.K. Rowling's *Harry Potter* series would be different than the audience for a biography of George Washington. The audience an author chooses to address is closely tied to the purpose of the work. The choice of an audience also drives the choice of language and level of diction an author uses. Ultimately, the intended audience determines the level to which that subject matter is presented and the complexity of the theme.

Author's Attitude in the Tone of a Passage

Style, tone, and mood are often thought to be the same thing. Although they're closely related, there are important differences to keep in mind. The easiest way to do this is to remember that style creates and affects tone and mood. More specifically, style is *how the writer uses words* to create the desired tone and mood for their writing.

Style

Style can include any number of technical writing choices, and some may have to be analyzed on the test. A few examples of style choices include:

- Sentence Construction: When presenting facts, does the writer use shorter sentences to create a quicker sense of the supporting evidence, or do they use longer sentences to elaborate and explain the information?

- Technical Language: Does the writer use jargon to demonstrate their expertise in the subject, or do they use ordinary language to help the reader understand things in simple terms?

- Formal Language: Does the writer refrain from using contractions such as *won't* or *can't* to create a more formal tone, or do they use a colloquial, conversational style to connect with the reader?

- Formatting: Does the writer use a series of shorter paragraphs to help the reader follow a line of argument, or do they use longer paragraphs to examine an issue in great detail and demonstrate their knowledge of the topic?

On the exam, test takers should examine the writer's style and how the author's writing choices affect the way that the text comes across.

Tone

Tone refers to the writer's attitude toward the subject matter. For example, the tone conveys how the writer feels about the topic he or she is writing about. A lot of nonfiction writing has a neutral tone, which is an important tone for the writer to take. A neutral tone demonstrates that the writer is presenting a topic impartially and letting the information speak for itself. On the other hand, nonfiction writing can be just as effective and appropriate if the tone isn't neutral. For instance, take this example:

> Seat belts save more lives than any other automobile safety feature. Many studies show that airbags save lives as well; however, not all cars have airbags. For instance, some older cars don't. Furthermore, air bags aren't entirely reliable. For example, studies show that in 15% of accidents airbags don't deploy as designed, but, on the other hand, seat belt malfunctions are extremely rare. The number of highway fatalities has plummeted since laws requiring seat belt usage were enacted.

In this passage, the writer mostly chooses to retain a neutral tone when presenting information. If the writer would instead include his or her own personal experience of losing a friend or family member in a car accident, the tone would change dramatically. The tone would no longer be neutral and would show that the writer has a personal stake in the content, allowing them to interpret the information in a different way. When analyzing tone, test takers should consider what the writer is trying to achieve in the text and how they *create* the tone using style.

Mood

Mood refers to the feelings and atmosphere that the writer's words create for the reader. Like tone, many nonfiction texts can have a neutral mood. To return to the previous example, if the writer would choose to include information about a person they know being killed in a car accident, the text would suddenly carry an emotional component that is absent in the previous example. Depending on how the writer presents the information, he or she can create a sad, angry, or even hopeful mood. When analyzing the mood, test takers should consider what the writer wants to accomplish and whether the best choice was made to achieve that end.

Identifying Literary Elements

There is no one, final definition of what literary elements are. They can be considered features or characteristics of fiction, but they are really more of a way that readers can unpack a text for the purpose of analysis and understanding the meaning. The elements contribute to a reader's literary interpretation of a passage as to how they function to convey the central message of a work. The most common literary elements used for analysis are the presented below.

Point of View
The *point of view* is the position the narrator takes when telling the story in prose. If a narrator is incorporated in a drama, the point of view may vary; in poetry, point of view refers to the position the speaker in a poem takes.

First Person
The first person point of view is when the writer uses the word "I" in the text. Poetry often uses first person, e.g., William Wordsworth's "I Wandered Lonely as a Cloud." Two examples of prose written in first person are Suzanne Collins' *The Hunger Games* and Anthony Burgess's *A Clockwork Orange*.

Second Person
The second person point of view is when the writer uses the pronoun "you." It is not widely used in prose fiction, but as a technique, it has been used by writers such as William Faulkner in *Absalom, Absalom!* and Albert Camus in *The Fall*. It is more common in poetry—e.g., Pablo Neruda's "If You Forget Me."

Third Person
Third person point of view is when the writer utilizes pronouns such as him, her, or them. It may be the most utilized point of view in prose as it provides flexibility to an author and is the one with which readers are most familiar. There are two main types of third person used in fiction. *Third person omniscient* uses a narrator that is all-knowing, relating the story by conveying and interpreting thoughts/feelings of all characters. In *third person limited,* the narrator relates the story through the perspective of one character's thoughts/feelings, usually the main character.

Plot
The *plot* is what happens in the story. Plots may be singular, containing one problem, or they may be very complex, with many sub-plots. All plots have exposition, a conflict, a climax, and a resolution. The *conflict* drives the plot and is something that the reader expects to be resolved. The plot carries those events along until there is a resolution to the conflict.

Tone
The *tone* of a story reflects the author's attitude and opinion about the subject matter of the story or text. Tone can be expressed through word choice, imagery, figurative language, syntax, and other details. The emotion or mood the reader experiences relates back to the tone of the story. Some examples of possible tones are humorous, somber, sentimental, and ironic.

Setting
The *setting* is the time, place, or set of surroundings in which the story occurs. It includes time or time span, place(s), climates, geography—man-made or natural—or cultural environments. Emily Dickinson's

poem "Because I could not stop for Death" has a simple setting—the narrator's symbolic ride with Death through town towards the local graveyard. Conversely, Leo Tolstoy's *War and Peace* encompasses numerous settings within settings in the areas affected by the Napoleonic Wars, spanning 1805 to 1812.

Characters

Characters are the story's figures that assume primary, secondary, or minor roles. *Central* or *major* characters are those integral to the story—the plot cannot be resolved without them. A central character can be a *protagonist* or hero. There may be more than one protagonist, and he/she doesn't always have to possess good characteristics. A character can also be an *antagonist*—the force against a protagonist.

Dynamic characters change over the course of the plot time. *Static* characters do not change. A *symbolic* character is one that represents an author's idea about society in general—e.g., Napoleon in Orwell's *Animal Farm*. *Stock* characters are those that appear across genres and embrace stereotypes—e.g., the cowboy of the Wild West or the blonde bombshell in a detective novel. A *flat* character is one that does not present a lot of complexity or depth, while a *rounded* character does. Sometimes, the *narrator* of a story or the *speaker* in a poem can be a character—e.g., Nick Carraway in F. Scott Fitzgerald's *The Great Gatsby* or the speaker in Robert Browning's "My Last Duchess." The narrator might also function as a character in prose, though not be part of the story—e.g., Charles Dickens' narrator of *A Christmas Carol*.

Understanding the Task, Purpose, and Audience

Identifying the Task, Purpose, and Intended Audience

An author's *writing style*—the way in which words, grammar, punctuation, and sentence fluidity are used—is the most influential element in a piece of writing, and it is dependent on the purpose and the audience for whom it is intended. Together, a writing style and mode of writing form the foundation of a written work, and a good writer will choose the most effective mode and style to convey a message to readers.

Writers should first determine what they are trying to say and then choose the most effective mode of writing to communicate that message. Different writing modes and *word choices* will affect the tone of a piece—that is, its underlying attitude, emotion, or character. The argumentative mode may utilize words that are earnest, angry, passionate, or excited whereas an informative piece may have a sterile, germane, or enthusiastic tone. The tones found in narratives vary greatly, depending on the purpose of the writing. *Tone* will also be affected by the audience—teaching science to children or those who may be uninterested would be most effective with enthusiastic language and exclamation points whereas teaching science to college students may take on a more serious and professional tone, with fewer charged words and punctuation choices that are inherent to academia.

Sentence fluidity—whether sentences are long and rhythmic or short and succinct—also affects a piece of writing as it determines the way in which a piece is read. Children or audiences unfamiliar with a subject do better with short, succinct sentence structures as these break difficult concepts up into shorter points. A period, question mark, or exclamation point is literally a signal for the reader to stop and takes more time to process. Thus, longer, more complex sentences are more appropriate for adults or educated audiences as they can fit more information in between processing time.

The amount of *supporting detail* provided is also tailored to the audience. A text that introduces a new subject to its readers will focus more on broad ideas without going into greater detail whereas a text that focuses on a more specific subject is likely to provide greater detail about the ideas discussed.

Writing styles, like modes, are most effective when tailored to their audiences. Having awareness of an audience's demographic is one of the most crucial aspects of properly communicating an argument, a story, or a set of information.

<u>Choosing the Most Appropriate Type of Writing</u>
Before beginning any writing, it is imperative that a writer have a firm grasp on the message he or she wishes to convey and how he or she wants readers to be affected by the writing. For example, does the author want readers to be more informed about the subject? Does the writer want readers to agree with his or her opinion? Does the writer want readers to get caught up in an exciting narrative? The following steps are a guide to determining the appropriate type of writing for a task, purpose, and audience:

1. Identifying the purpose for writing the piece
2. Determining the audience
3. Adapting the writing mode, word choices, tone, and style to fit the audience and the purpose

It is important to distinguish between a work's purpose and its main idea. The essential difference between the two is that the *main idea* is what the author wants to communicate about the topic at hand whereas the *primary purpose* is why the author is writing in the first place. The primary purpose is what will determine the type of writing an author will choose to utilize, not the main idea, though the two are related. For example, if an author writes an article on the mistreatment of animals in factory farms and, at the end, suggests that people should convert to vegetarianism, the main idea is that vegetarianism would reduce the poor treatment of animals. The primary purpose is to convince the reader to stop eating animals. Since the primary purpose is to galvanize an audience into action, the author would choose the argumentative writing mode.

The next step is to consider to whom the author is appealing as this will determine the type of details to be included, the diction to be used, the tone to be employed, and the sentence structure to be used. An audience can be identified by considering the following questions:

- What is the purpose for writing the piece?

- To whom is it being written?

- What is their age range?

- Are they familiar with the material being presented, or are they just being newly introduced to it?

- Where are they from?

- Is the task at hand in a professional or casual setting?

- Is the task at hand for monetary gain?

These are just a few of the numerous considerations to keep in mind, but the main idea is to become as familiar with the audience as possible. Once the audience has been understood, the author can then adapt the writing style to align with the readers' education and interests. The audience is what determines the *rhetorical appeal* the author will use—ethos, pathos, or logos. *Ethos* is a rhetorical appeal to an audience's ethics and/or morals. Ethos is most often used in argumentative and informative writing modes. *Pathos* is an appeal to the audience's emotions and sympathies, and it is found in argumentative, descriptive, and narrative writing modes. *Logos* is an appeal to the audience's logic and reason and is used primarily in informative texts as well as in supporting details for argumentative pieces. Rhetorical appeals are discussed in depth in the informational texts and rhetoric section of the test.

If the author is trying to encourage global conversion to vegetarianism, he or she may choose to use all three rhetorical appeals to reach varying personality types. Those who are less interested in the welfare of animals but are interested in facts and science would relate more to logos. Animal lovers would relate better to an emotional appeal. In general, the most effective works utilize all three appeals.

Finally, after determining the writing mode and rhetorical appeal, the author will consider word choice, sentence structure, and tone, depending on the purpose and audience. The author may choose words that convey sadness or anger when speaking about animal welfare if writing to persuade, or he or she will stick to dispassionate and matter-of-fact tones, if informing the public on the treatment of animals in factory farms. If the author is writing to a younger or less-educated audience, he or she may choose to shorten and simplify sentence structures and word choice. If appealing to an audience with more expert knowledge on a particular subject, writers will more likely employ a style of longer sentences and more complex vocabulary.

Depending on the task, the author may choose to use a first person, second person, or third person point of view. First person and second person perspectives are inherently more casual in tone, including the author and the reader in the rhetoric, while third person perspectives are often seen in more professional settings.

Evaluating the Effectiveness of a Piece of Writing
An effective and engaging piece of writing will cause the reader to forget about the author entirely. Readers will become so engrossed in the subject, argument, or story at hand that they will almost identify with it, readily adopting beliefs proposed by the author or accepting all elements of the story as believable. On the contrary, poorly written works will cause the reader to be hyperaware of the author, doubting the writer's knowledge of a subject or questioning the validity of a narrative. Persuasive or expository works that are poorly researched will have this effect, as well as poorly planned stories with significant plot holes. An author must consider the task, purpose, and audience to sculpt a piece of writing effectively.

When evaluating the effectiveness of a piece, the most important thing to consider is how well the purpose is conveyed to the audience through the mode, use of rhetoric, and writing style.

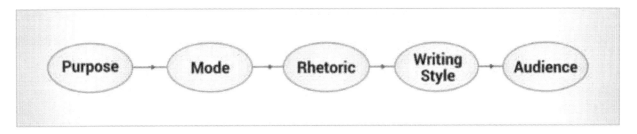

The purpose must pass through these three aspects for effective delivery to the audience. If any elements are not properly considered, the reader will be overly aware of the author, and the message will be lost. The following is a checklist for evaluating the effectiveness of a piece:

- Does the writer choose the appropriate writing mode—argumentative, narrative, descriptive, informative—for his or her purpose?

- Does the writing mode employed contain characteristics inherent to that mode?

- Does the writer consider the personalities/interests/demographics of the intended audience when choosing rhetorical appeals?

- Does the writer use appropriate vocabulary, sentence structure, voice, and tone for the audience demographic?

- Does the author properly establish himself/herself as having authority on the subject, if applicable?

- Does the piece make sense?

Another thing to consider is the medium in which the piece was written. If the medium is a blog, diary, or personal letter, the author may adopt a more casual stance towards the audience. If the piece of writing is a story in a book, a business letter or report, or a published article in a journal or if the task is to gain money or support or to get published, the author may adopt a more formal stance. Ultimately, the writer will want to be very careful in how he or she addresses the reader.

Finally, the effectiveness of a piece can be evaluated by asking how well the purpose was achieved. For example, if students are assigned to read a persuasive essay, instructors can ask whether the author influences students' opinions. Students may be assigned two differing persuasive texts with opposing perspectives and be asked which writer was more convincing. Students can then evaluate what factors contributed to this—for example, whether one author uses more credible supporting facts, appeals more effectively to readers' emotions, presents more believable personal anecdotes, or offers stronger counterargument refutation. Students can then use these evaluations to strengthen their own writing skills.

Identifying Major Literary Works and Authors

In most cases on the MCAT, the test taker will be presented with a passage and be required to answer one or more questions about it. The ability of the test taker to demonstrate familiarity of major literary works is helpful on the MCAT, though it is not required. The following chart offers some examples of major works in addition to those listed elsewhere in this guide, but the list not exhaustive.

American
Fictional Prose Before 1920
- Nathaniel Hawthorne | *The Scarlett Letter* (1850)
- Harriet Beecher Stowe | *Uncle Tom's Cabin* (1852)
- Louisa May Alcott | *Little Women* (1868)
- Henry James | *Daisy Miller* (1878)
- Jack London | *The Call of the Wild* (1903)
- William Faulkner | *The Sound and the Fury* (1929)

Fictional Prose After 1920 and Before 1960
- Zora Neale Hurston | *Their Eyes Were Watching God* (1937)
- John Steinbeck | *Grapes of Wrath* (1939)
- Ernest Hemingway | *For Whom the Bell Tolls* (1940)
- J.D. Salinger | *Catcher in the Rye* (1951)
- Herman Melville | *Moby Dick* (1956)

Fictional Prose After 1960
- Harper Lee | *To Kill a Mockingbird* (1960)
- N. Scott Momaday | *The Way to Rainy Mountain* (1969)
- Marilynne Robinson | *Housekeeping* (1980)
- Alice Walker | *The Color Purple* (1982)
- Toni Morrison | *Beloved* (1987)

Drama
- Thornton Wilder I *Our Town* (1938)
- Tennessee Williams | *A Streetcar Named Desire* (1947)
- Eugene O'Neill |*Long Day's Journey into Night* (1956)
- Lorraine Hansberry | *A Raisin in the Sun* (1959)
- Edward Albee | *Who's Afraid of Virginia Woolf?* (1962)
- Amiri Baraka | *Dutchman* (1964)
- Sam Shephard | *Buried Child* (1978)

Poetry
- Anne Bradstreet | "In Reference to her Children, 23 June 1659"
- Phillis Wheatley | "On Being Brought from Africa to America" (1768)
- Edgar Allen Poe | "The Raven" (1845)
- Walt Whitman | "Song of Myself" (1855)
- Emily Dickinson | "Because I could not stop for Death" (1863)
- Robert Frost | "Wild Grapes" (1920)
- Langston Hughes | "Harlem" (1951)
- Richard Wilbur | "Love Calls Us to the Things of This World" (1956)
- Sylvia Plath | "Mirror" (1961)
- Eamon Grennan | "Cat Scat" (1988)
- Sandra Cisneros | "Loose Woman" (1994)
- Anne Carson | "The Glass Essay" (1994)
- Tupac Shakur | "The Rose that Grew from Concrete" (1999)

Literary Non-fiction
- Frederick Douglass | *My Bondage and My Freedom* (1855)
- Anne Frank | *The Diary of Anne Frank* (1947)
- Truman Capote | *In Cold Blood* (1966)
- Maya Angelou | *I Know Why the Caged Bird Sings* (1969)
- Sherman Alexie | *The Absolutely True Diary of a Part-Time Indian* (2007)
- Cynthia Levinson | *We've Got a Job* (2012)
- Malala Yousafzai and Christina Lamb | *I am Malala* (2013)
- Philip Hoose | *The Boys who Challenged Hitler* (2015

Identifying Literary Contexts

Understanding that works of literature emerged either because of a particular context—or perhaps despite a context—is key to analyzing them effectively.

Historical Context
The *historical context* of a piece of literature can refer to the time period, setting, or conditions of living at the time it was written as well as the context of the work. For example, Hawthorne's *The Scarlet Letter* was published in 1850, though the setting of the story is 1642-1649. Historically, then, when Hawthorne wrote his novel, the United States found itself at odds as the beginnings of a potential Civil War were in view. Thus, the historical context is potentially significant as it pertains to the ideas of traditions and values, which Hawthorne addresses in his story of Hester Prynne in the era of Puritanism.

Cultural Context
The *cultural context* of a piece of literature refers to cultural factors, such as the beliefs, religions, and customs that surround and are in a work of literature. The Puritan's beliefs, religion, and customs in Hawthorne's novel would be significant as they are at the core of the plot—the reason Hester wears the A and why Arthur kills himself. The customs of people in the Antebellum Period, though not quite as restrictive, were still somewhat similar. This would impact how the audience of the time received the novel.

Literary Context
Literary context refers to the consideration of the genre, potentially at the time the work was written. In 1850, Realism and Romanticism were the driving forces in literature in the U.S., with depictions of life as it was at the time in which the work was written or the time it was written *about* as well as some works celebrating the beauty of nature. Thus, an audience in Hawthorne's time would have been well satisfied with the elements of both offered in the text. They would have been looking for details about everyday things and people (Realism), but they also would appreciate his approach to description of nature and the focus on the individual (American Romanticism). The contexts would be significant as they would pertain to evaluating the work against those criteria.

Here are some questions to use when considering context:

- When was the text written?
- What was society like at the time the text was written, or what was it like, given the work's identified time period?
- Who or what influenced the writer?
- What political or social influences might there have been?
- What influences may there have been in the genre that may have affected the writer?

Additionally, test takers should familiarize themselves with literary periods such as Old and Middle English, American Colonial, American Renaissance, American Naturalistic, and British and American Modernist and Post-Modernist movements. Most students of literature will have had extensive exposure to these literary periods in history, and while it is not necessary to recognize every major literary work on sight and associate that work to its corresponding movement or cultural context, the test taker should be familiar enough with the historical and cultural significance of each test passage in order to be able to address test questions correctly.

The following brief description of some literary contexts and their associated literary examples follows. It is not an all-inclusive list. The test taker should read each description, then follow up with independent study to clarify each movement, its context, its most familiar authors, and their works.

Metaphysical Poetry

Metaphysical poetry is the descriptor applied to 17th century poets whose poetry emphasized the lyrical quality of their work. These works contain highly creative poetic conceits or metaphoric comparisons between two highly dissimilar things or ideas. Metaphysical poetry is characterized by highly prosaic language and complicated, often layered, metaphor.

Poems such as John Donne's "The Flea," Andrew Marvell's "To His Coy Mistress," George Herbert's "The Collar," Henry Vaughan's "The World," and Richard Crashaw's "A Song" are associated with this type of poetry.

British Romanticism

British Romanticism was a cultural and literary movement within Europe that developed at the end of the 18th century and extended into the 19th century. It occurred partly in response to aristocratic, political, and social norms and partly in response to the Industrial Revolution of the day. Characterized by intense emotion, major literary works of British Romanticism embrace the idea of aestheticism and the beauty of nature. Literary works exalted folk customs and historical art and encouraged spontaneity of artistic endeavor. The movement embraced the heroic ideal and the concept that heroes would raise the quality of society.

Authors who are classified as British Romantics include Samuel Taylor Coleridge, John Keats, George Byron, Mary Shelley, Percy Bysshe Shelley, and William Blake. Well-known works include Samuel Taylor Coleridge's "Kubla Khan," John Keats' "Ode on a Grecian Urn," George Byron's "Childe Harold's Pilgrimage," Mary Shelley's *Frankenstein*, Percy Bysshe Shelley's "Ode to the West Wind," and William Blake's "The Tyger."

American Romanticism

American Romanticism occurred within the American literary scene beginning early in the 19th century. While many aspects were similar to British Romanticism, it is further characterized as having gothic aspects and the idea that individualism was to be encouraged. It also embraced the concept of the *noble savage*—the idea that indigenous culture uncorrupted by civilization is better than advanced society.

Well-known authors and works include Nathanial Hawthorne's *The House of the Seven Gables*, Edgar Allan Poe's "The Raven" and "The Cask of Amontillado," Emily Dickinson's "I Felt a Funeral in My Brain" and James Fenimore Cooper's *The Last of the Mohicans*.

Transcendentalism

Transcendentalism was a movement that applied to a way of thinking that developed within the United States, specifically New England, around 1836. While this way of thinking originally employed philosophical aspects, transcendentalism spread to all forms of art, literature, and even to the ways people chose to live. It was born out of a reaction to traditional rationalism and purported concepts such as a higher divinity, feminism, humanitarianism, and communal living. Transcendentalism valued intuition, self-reliance, and the idea that human nature was inherently good.

Well-known authors include Ralph Waldo Emerson, Henry David Thoreau, Louisa May Alcott, and Ellen Sturgis Hooper. Works include Ralph Waldo Emerson's "Self-Reliance" and "Uriel," Henry David

Thoreau's *Walden* and *Civil Disobedience*, Louisa May Alcott's *Little Women*, and Ellen Sturgis Hooper's "I Slept, and Dreamed that Life was Beauty."

The Harlem Renaissance

The Harlem Renaissance is the descriptor given to the cultural, artistic, and social boom that developed in Harlem, New York, at the beginning of the 20ᵗʰ century, spanning the 1920s and 1930s. Originally termed *The New Negro Movement*, it emphasized African-American urban cultural expression and migration across the United States. It had strong roots in African-American Christianity, discourse, and intellectualism. The Harlem Renaissance heavily influenced the development of music and fashion as well. Its singular characteristic was to embrace Pan-American culturalisms; however, strong themes of the slavery experience and African-American folk traditions also emerged. A hallmark of the Harlem Renaissance was that it laid the foundation for the future Civil Rights Movement in the United States.

Well-known authors and works include Zora Neale Hurston's *Their Eyes Were Watching God*, Richard Wright's *Native Son*, Langston Hughes' "I, Too," and James Weldon Johnson's "God's Trombones: Seven Negro Sermons in Verse" and *The Book of American Negro Poetry*.

Understanding the Characteristics of Literary Genres

Classifying literature involves an understanding of the concept of genre. A *genre* is a category of literature that possesses similarities in style and in characteristics. Based on form and structure, there are four basic genres.

Fictional Prose

Fictional prose consists of fictional works written in standard form with a natural flow of speech and without poetic structure. Fictional prose primarily utilizes grammatically complete sentences and a paragraph structure to convey its message.

Drama

Drama is fiction that is written to be performed in a variety of media, intended to be performed for an audience, and structured for that purpose. It might be composed using poetry or prose, often straddling the elements of both in what actors are expected to present. Action and dialogue are the tools used in drama to tell the story.

Poetry

Poetry is fiction in verse that has a unique focus on the rhythm of language and focuses on intensity of feeling. It is not an entire story, though it may tell one; it is compact in form and in function. Poetry can be considered as a poet's brief word picture for a reader. Poetic structure is primarily composed of lines and stanzas. Together, poetic structure and devices are the methods that poets use to lead readers to feeling an effect and, ultimately, to the interpretive message.

Literary Nonfiction

Literary nonfiction is prose writing that is based on current or past real events or real people and includes straightforward accounts as well as those that offer opinions on facts or factual events. The MCAT exam distinguishes between *literary nonfiction*—a form of writing that incorporates literary styles and techniques to create factually-based narratives—and informational texts.

Biography

A *biography* is a work written about a real person (historical or currently living). It involves factual accounts of the person's life, often in a re-telling of those events based on available, researched factual information. The re-telling and dialogue, especially if related within quotes, must be accurate and reflect reliable sources. A biography reflects the time and place in which the person lived, with the goal of creating an understanding of the person and his/her human experience. Examples of well-known biographies include *The Life of Samuel Johnson* by James Boswell and *Steve Jobs* by Walter Isaacson.

Autobiography

An *autobiography* is a factual account of a person's life written by that person. It may contain some or all of the same elements as a biography, but the author is the subject matter. An autobiography will be told in first person narrative. Examples of well-known autobiographies in literature include *Night* by Elie Wiesel and *Margaret Thatcher: The Autobiography* by Margaret Thatcher.

Memoir

A *memoir* is a historical account of a person's life and experiences written by one who has personal, intimate knowledge of the information. The line between memoir, autobiography, and biography is often muddled, but generally speaking, a memoir covers a specific timeline of events as opposed to the other forms of nonfiction. A memoir is less all-encompassing. It is also less formal in tone and tends to focus on the emotional aspect of the presented timeline of events. Some examples of memoirs in literature include *Angela's Ashes* by Frank McCourt and *All Creatures Great and Small* by James Herriot.

Journalism

Some forms of *journalism* can fall into the category of literary non-fiction—e.g., travel writing, nature writing, sports writing, the interview, and sometimes, the essay. Some examples include Elizabeth Kolbert's "The Lost World, in the Annals of Extinction series for *The New Yorker* and Gary Smith's "Ali and His Entourage" for ***Sports Illustrated***.

Informational Texts

Informational texts are a category of texts within the genre of nonfiction. Their intent is to inform, and while they do convey a point of view and may include literary devices, they do not utilize other literary elements, such as characters or plot. An informational text also reflects a *thesis*—an implicit or explicit statement of the text's intent and/or a *main idea*—the overarching focus and/or purpose of the text, generally implied. Some examples of informational texts are informative articles, instructional/how-to texts, factual reports, reference texts, and self-help texts.

Interpreting Textual Evidence in Informational Text
Literal and Figurative Meanings
It is important when evaluating informational texts to consider the use of both literal and figurative meanings. The words and phrases an author chooses to include in a text must be evaluated. How does the word choice affect the meaning and tone? By recognizing the use of literal and figurative language, a reader can more readily ascertain the message or purpose of a text. Literal word choice is the easiest to analyze as it represents the usual and intended way a word or phrase is used. It is also more common in informational texts because it is used to state facts and definitions. While figurative language is typically associated with fiction and poetry, it can be found in informational texts as well. The reader must

determine not only what is meant by the figurative language in context, but also how the author intended it to shape the overall text.

Inference in Informational Text
Inference refers to the reader's ability to understand the unwritten text, i.e., "read between the lines" in terms of an author's intent or message. The strategy asks that a reader not take everything he or she reads at face value but instead, add his or her own interpretation of what the author seems to be trying to convey. A reader's ability to make inferences relies on his or her ability to think clearly and logically about the text. It does not ask that the reader make wild speculation or guess about the material but demands that he or she be able to come to a sound conclusion about the material.

An author's use of less literal words and phrases requires readers to make more inference when they read. Since inference involves *deduction*—deriving conclusions from ideas assumed to be true—there's more room for interpretation. Still, critical readers who employ inference, if careful in their thinking, can still arrive at the logical, sound conclusions the author intends.

Textual Evidence in Informational Text
Once a reader has determined an author's thesis or main idea, he or she will need to understand how textual evidence supports interpretation of that thesis or main idea. Test takers will be asked direct questions regarding an author's main idea and may be asked to identify evidence that would support those ideas. This will require test takers to comprehend literal and figurative meanings within the text passage, be able to draw inferences from provided information, and be able to separate important evidence from minor supporting detail. It's often helpful to skim test questions and answer options prior to critically reading informational text; however, test takers should avoid the temptation to solely look for the correct answers. Just trying to find the "right answer" may cause test takers to miss important supporting textual evidence. Making mental note of test questions is only helpful as a guide when reading.

After identifying an author's thesis or main idea, a test taker should look at the supporting details that the author provides to back up his or her assertions, identifying those additional pieces of information that help expand the thesis. From there, test takers should examine that additional information and related details for credibility, the author's use of outside sources, and be able to point to direct evidence that supports the author's claims. It's also imperative that test takers be able to identify what is strong support and what is merely additional information that is nice to know but not necessary. Being able to make this differentiation will help test takers effectively answer questions regarding an author's use of supporting evidence within informational text.

Understanding Organizational Patterns and Structures
Organizational Structure within Informational Text
Informational text is specifically designed to relate factual information, and although it is open to a reader's interpretation and application of the facts, the structure of the presentation is carefully designed to lead the reader to a particular conclusion or central idea. When reading informational text, it is important that readers are able to understand its organizational structure as the structure often directly relates to an author's intent to inform and/or persuade the reader.

The first step in identifying the text's structure is to determine the thesis or main idea. The thesis statement and organization of a work are closely intertwined. *A thesis statement* indicates the writer's purpose and may include the scope and direction of the text. It may be presented at the beginning of a text or at the end, and it may be explicit or implicit.

Once a reader has a grasp of the thesis or main idea of the text, he or she can better determine its organizational structure. Test takers are advised to read informational text passages more than once in order to comprehend the material fully. It is also helpful to examine any text features present in the text including the table of contents, index, glossary, headings, footnotes, and visuals. The analysis of these features and the information presented within them, can offer additional clues about the central idea and structure of a text. The following questions should be asked when considering structure:

- How does the author assemble the parts to make an effective whole argument?
- Is the passage linear in nature and if so, what is the timeline or thread of logic?
- What is the presented order of events, facts, or arguments? Are these effective in contributing to the author's thesis?
- How can the passage be divided into sections? How are they related to each other and to the main idea or thesis?
- What key terms are used to indicate the organization?

Next, test takers should skim the passage, noting the first line or two of each body paragraph—the *topic sentences*—and the conclusion. Key *transitional terms*, such as *on the other hand, also, because, however, therefore, most importantly*, and *first*, within the text can also signal organizational structure. Based on these clues, readers should then be able to identify what type of organizational structure is being used. The following organizational structures are most common:

- *Problem/solution*—organized by an analysis/overview of a problem, followed by potential solution(s)

- *Cause/effect*—organized by the effects resulting from a cause or the cause(s) of a particular effect

- *Spatial order*—organized by points that suggest location or direction—e.g., top to bottom, right to left, outside to inside

- *Chronological/sequence order*—organized by points presented to indicate a passage of time or through purposeful steps/stages

- *Comparison/Contrast*—organized by points that indicate similarities and/or differences between two things or concepts

- *Order of importance*—organized by priority of points, often most significant to least significant or vice versa

Rhetorical Devices, Word Choice, and Text Structure

Identifying Rhetorical Devices

If one feels strongly about a subject, or has a passion for it, they choose strong words and phrases. Think of the types of rhetoric (or language) our politicians use. Each word, phrase, and idea is carefully crafted to elicit a response. Hopefully, that response is one of agreement to a certain point of view, especially among voters. Authors use the same types of language to achieve the same results. For example, the word "bad" has a certain connotation, but the words "horrid," "repugnant," and "abhorrent" paint a far better picture for the reader. They're more precise. They're interesting to read and they should all illicit stronger feelings in the reader than the word "bad." An author generally uses other devices beyond mere word choice to persuade, convince, entertain, or otherwise engage a reader.

Rhetorical devices are those elements an author utilizes in painting sensory, and hopefully persuasive ideas to which a reader can relate. They are numerable. Test takers will likely encounter one or more standardized test questions addressing varying rhetorical devices. This study guide will address the more common types: alliteration, irony, metaphor, simile, hyperbole, allegory, imagery, onomatopoeia, and personification, providing examples of each.

Alliteration is a device that uses repetitive beginning sounds in words to appeal to the reader. Classic tongue twisters are a great example of alliteration. *She sells sea shells down by the sea shore* is an extreme example of alliteration. Authors will use alliterative devices to capture a reader's attention. It's interesting to note that marketing also utilizes alliteration in the same way. A reader will likely remember products that have the brand name and item starting with the same letter. Similarly, many songs, poems, and catchy phrases use this device. It's memorable. Use of alliteration draws a reader's attention to ideas that an author wants to highlight.

Irony is a device that authors use when pitting two contrasting items or ideas against each other in order to create an effect. It's frequently used when an author wants to employ humor or convey a sarcastic tone. Additionally, it's often used in fictional works to build tension between characters, or between a particular character and the reader. An author may use *verbal irony* (sarcasm), *situational irony* (where actions or events have the opposite effect than what's expected), and *dramatic irony* (where the reader knows something a character does not). Examples of irony include:

- Dramatic Irony: An author describing the presence of a hidden killer in a murder mystery, unbeknownst to the characters but known to the reader.

- Situational Irony: An author relating the tale of a fire captain who loses her home in a five-alarm conflagration.

- Verbal Irony: This is where an author or character says one thing but means another. For example, telling a police officer "Thanks a lot" after receiving a ticket.

Metaphor is a device that uses a figure of speech to paint a visual picture of something that is not literally applicable. Authors relate strong images to readers, and evoke similar strong feelings using metaphors. Most often, authors will mention one thing in comparison to another more familiar to the reader. It's important to note that metaphors do not use the comparative words "like" or "as." At times, metaphors encompass common phrases such as clichés. At other times, authors may use mixed metaphors in making identification between two dissimilar things. Examples of metaphors include:

- An author describing a character's anger as *a flaming sheet of fire.*
- An author relating a politician as having been a folding chair under close questioning.
- A novel's character telling another character to *take a flying hike.*
- Shakespeare's assertion that *all the world's a stage.*

Simile is a device that compares two dissimilar things using the words "like" and "as." When using similes, an author tries to catch a reader's attention and use comparison of unlike items to make a point. Similes are commonly used and often develop into figures of speech and catch phrases.

Examples of similes include:

- An author describing a character as having a complexion like a faded lily.

- An investigative journalist describing his interview subject as being like cold steel and with a demeanor hard as ice.

- An author asserting the current political arena is just like a three-ring circus and as dry as day old bread.

Similes and metaphors can be confusing. When utilizing simile, an author will state one thing is like another. A metaphor states one thing is another. An example of the difference would be if an author states a character is *just like a fierce tiger and twice as angry,* as opposed to stating the character *is a fierce tiger and twice as angry.*

Hyperbole is simply an exaggeration that is not taken literally. A potential test taker will have heard or employed hyperbole in daily speech, as it is a common device we all use. Authors will use hyperbole to draw a reader's eye toward important points and to illicit strong emotional and relatable responses. Examples of hyperbole include:

- An author describing a character as being as big as a house and twice the circumference of a city block.

- An author stating the city's water problem as being old as the hills and more expensive than a king's ransom in spent tax dollars.

- A journalist stating the mayoral candidate died of embarrassment when her tax records were made public.

Allegories are stories or poems with hidden meanings, usually a political or moral one. Authors will frequently use allegory when leading the reader to a conclusion. Allegories are similar to parables, symbols, and analogies. Often, an author will employ the use of allegory to make political, historical, moral, or social observations. As an example, Jonathan Swift's work *Gulliver's Travels into Several Remote Nations of the World* is an allegory in and of itself. The work is a political allegory of England during Jonathan Swift's lifetime. Set in the travel journal style plot of a giant amongst smaller people, and a smaller Gulliver amongst the larger, it is a commentary on Swift's political stance of existing issues of his age. Many fictional works are entire allegories in and of themselves. George Orwell's *Animal Farm* is a story of animals that conquer man and form their own farm society with swine at the top; however, it is not a literal story in any sense. It's Orwell's political allegory of Russian society during and after the Communist revolution of 1917. Other examples of allegory in popular culture include:

- Aesop's fable "The Tortoise and the Hare," which teaches readers that being steady is more important than being fast and impulsive.

- The popular *Hunger Games* by Suzanne Collins that teaches readers that media can numb society to what is truly real and important.

- Dr. Seuss's *Yertle the Turtle* which is a warning against totalitarianism and, at the time it was written, against the despotic rule of Adolf Hitler.

Imagery is a rhetorical device that an author employs when they use visual, or descriptive, language to evoke a reader's emotion. Use of imagery as a rhetorical device is broader in scope than this study guide addresses, but in general, the function of imagery is to create a vibrant scene in the reader's imagination and, in turn, tease the reader's ability to identify through strong emotion and sensory experience. In the simplest of terms, imagery, as a rhetoric device, beautifies literature.

An example of poetic imagery is below:

> Pain has an element of blank
>
> It cannot recollect
>
> When it began, or if there were
>
> A day when it was not.
>
> It has no future but itself,
>
> Its infinite realms contain
>
> Its past, enlightened to perceive
>
> New periods of pain.

In the above poem, Emily Dickenson uses strong imagery. Pain is equivalent to an "element of blank" or of nothingness. Pain cannot recollect a beginning or end, as if it was a person (see *personification* below). Dickenson appeals to the reader's sense of a painful experience by discussing the unlikelihood that discomfort sees a future, but does visualize a past and present. She simply indicates that pain, through the use of imagery, is cyclical and never ending. Dickenson's theme is one of painful depression and it is through the use of imagery that she conveys this to her readers.

Onomatopoeia is the author's use of words that create sound. Words like *pop* and *sizzle* are examples of onomatopoeia. When an author wants to draw a reader's attention in an auditory sense, they will use onomatopoeia. An author may also use onomatopoeia to create sounds as interjection or commentary. Examples include:

- An author describing a cat's vocalization as the kitten's chirrup echoed throughout the empty cabin.
- A description of a campfire as crackling and whining against its burning green wood.
- An author relating the sound of a car accident as *metallic screeching against crunching asphalt*.
- A description of an animal roadblock as being *a symphonic melody of groans, baas, and moans*.

Personification is a rhetorical device that an author uses to attribute human qualities to inanimate objects or animals. Once again, this device is useful when an author wants the reader to strongly relate to an idea. As in the example of George Orwell's *Animal Farm*, many of the animals are given the human abilities to speak, reason, apply logic, and otherwise interact as humans do. This helps the reader see how easily it is for any society to segregate into the haves and the have-nots through the manipulation of power. Personification is a device that enables the reader to empathize through human experience.

Examples of personification include:

- An author describing the wind as *whispering through the trees*.

- A description of a stone wall as being a hardened, unmovable creature made of cement and brick.

- An author attributing a city building as having slit eyes and an unapproachable, foreboding façade.

- An author describing spring as a beautiful bride, blooming in white, ready for summer's matrimony.

When identifying rhetorical devices, look for words and phrases that capture one's attention. Make note of the author's use of comparison between the inanimate and the animate. Consider words that make the reader feel sounds and envision imagery. Pay attention to the rhythm of fluid sentences and to the use of words that evoke emotion. The ability to identify rhetorical devices is another step in achieving successful reading comprehension and in being able to correctly answer standardized questions related to those devices.

Rhetorical Appeals

In nonfiction writing, authors employ argumentative techniques to present their opinion to readers in the most convincing way. First of all, persuasive writing usually includes at least one type of appeal: an appeal to logic (logos), emotion (pathos), or credibility and trustworthiness (ethos). When writers appeal to logic, they are asking readers to agree with them based on research, evidence, and an established line of reasoning. An author's argument might also appeal to readers' emotions, perhaps by including personal stories and anecdotes (a short narrative of a specific event). A final type of appeal, appeal to authority, asks the reader to agree with the author's argument on the basis of their expertise or credentials. Consider three different approaches to arguing the same opinion:

Logic (Logos)
Below is an example of an appeal to logic. The author uses evidence to disprove the logic of the school's rule (the rule was supposed to reduce discipline problems; the number of problems has not been reduced; therefore, the rule is not working) and call for its repeal.

> Our school should abolish its current ban on cell phone use on campus. This rule was adopted last year as an attempt to reduce class disruptions and help students focus more on their lessons. However, since the rule was enacted, there has been no change in the number of disciplinary problems in class. Therefore, the rule is ineffective and should be done away with.

Emotion (Pathos)
An author's argument might also appeal to readers' emotions, perhaps by including personal stories and anecdotes. The next example presents an appeal to emotion. By sharing the personal anecdote of one student and speaking about emotional topics like family relationships, the author invokes the reader's empathy in asking them to reconsider the school rule.

> Our school should abolish its current ban on cell phone use on campus. If they aren't able to use their phones during the school day, many students feel isolated from their loved ones. For example, last semester, one student's grandmother had a heart attack in the morning. However,

because he couldn't use his cell phone, the student didn't know about his grandmother's accident until the end of the day—when she had already passed away and it was too late to say goodbye. By preventing students from contacting their friends and family, our school is placing undue stress and anxiety on students.

Credibility (Ethos)

Finally, an appeal to authority includes a statement from a relevant expert. In this case, the author uses a doctor in the field of education to support the argument. All three examples begin from the same opinion—the school's phone ban needs to change—but rely on different argumentative styles to persuade the reader.

> Our school should abolish its current ban on cell phone use on campus. According to Dr. Bartholomew Everett, a leading educational expert, "Research studies show that cell phone usage has no real impact on student attentiveness. Rather, phones provide a valuable technological resource for learning. Schools need to learn how to integrate this new technology into their curriculum." Rather than banning phones altogether, our school should follow the advice of experts and allow students to use phones as part of their learning.

Rhetorical Questions

Another commonly used argumentative technique is asking rhetorical questions—questions that do not actually require an answer but that push the reader to consider the topic further.

> I wholly disagree with the proposal to ban restaurants from serving foods with high sugar and sodium contents. Do we really want to live in a world where the government can control what we eat? I prefer to make my own food choices.

Here, the author's rhetorical question prompts readers to put themselves in a hypothetical situation and imagine how they would feel about it.

Information that is Explicitly Stated

Readers want to draw a conclusion about what the author has presented. Drawing a conclusion will help the reader to understand what the writer intended as well as whether he or she agrees with what the author has said. There are a few ways to determine the logical conclusion, but careful reading is the most important. The passage should be read a few times, and readers should highlight or take notes on the details that they deem important to the meaning of the piece. Readers may draw a conclusion that is different than what the writer intended, or they may draw more than one conclusion. Readers should look carefully at the details to see if their conclusion matches up with what the writer has presented and intended for readers to understand. Of course, test takers may not have time to take notes or compare on the test itself. However, it may be helpful for test takers to practice this to make sure their comprehension skills are strong.

Textual evidence can help readers to draw a conclusion about a passage. Textual evidence refers to information such as facts and examples that support the main point. Textual evidence will likely come from outside sources, and can be in the form of quoted or paraphrased material. Readers should look to this evidence and its credibility and validity in relation to the main idea to draw a conclusion about the writing.

The author may state the conclusion directly in the passage. Inferring the author's conclusion is useful, especially when it is not overtly stated, but inferences should not outweigh the information that is directly stated. Alternatively, when readers are trying to draw a conclusion about a text, it may not always be directly stated.

As mentioned before, summary is another effective way to draw a conclusion from a passage. Summary is a shortened version of the original text, written in one's own words. It should focus on the main points of the original text, including only the relevant details. It's important to be brief but thorough in a summary. While the summary should always be shorter than the original passage, it should still retain the meaning of the original source.

Like summary, paraphrasing can also help a reader to fully understand a part of a reading. Paraphrase calls for the reader to take a small part of the passage and to say it in their own words. Paraphrase is more than rewording the original passage, though. It should be written in one's own way, while still retaining the meaning of the original source. When a reader's goal is to write something in their own words, deeper understanding of the original source is required. Again, applying summary and paraphrase to the passages during the test may not be the most efficient use of the test taker's time. However, these tools should be considered when one is practicing comprehending passages. Test takers who are familiar with carefully selecting important aspects of the passage will benefit from this experience on test day.

Information or Ideas that can be Inferred

Inference questions require drawing a conclusion using reasoning and evidence. Making an inference requires careful reading of the passage to determine the author's intended meaning. The author's main idea or overall meaning may be directly stated in the passage, but in some cases, it is not. The implied meaning is, by definition, not explicitly stated in the passage, so it is necessary for readers to use details from the passage to decipher the author's implications. It is possible for readers to draw a logical conclusion about the author's intended meaning by using the facts and evidence presented in the passage.

The Premise
Inference questions are based on the premises provided in the passage. Premises are the facts or evidence presented by the author. These premises should be taken as fact, even if they are based on the author's opinion. In some cases, the reader may disagree with the premises presented, or even know them to be untrue, but it is important to view the premises as fact. This is what the author believes and wants the reader to believe, so the premises will help lead the reader to the most logical conclusion.

There are certain clue words that can indicate the premises in a passage. These clue words include:

- because
- for
- since
- as
- given that
- in that
- as indicated by
- owing to

While these words can help the reader discover the author's premises, making an inference requires reading between the lines to find the implied meaning of the passage. The implications of the facts are what lead the reader to a logical conclusion.

Question Types
An inference question may focus on a word's meaning or ask the reader to draw a conclusion based on the evidence presented. It is helpful for readers to know that a question calls for inference, so it is not confused with assumption.

Some clues to look for are questions that use statements like the following:

- If the previous statements are true, it logically follows that
- Must be true
- Author's conclusion
- Best supported by

It's important for test takers to remember that the facts presented should be taken as true, even if they aren't. When answering this type of question, answers that could be true, but not based on the facts presented in the passage, should be avoided. Instead, readers should look for the only answer that must be true based on the premises provided. Test takers should also avoid making assumptions, as this is a different type of question. Making an inference is about drawing a logical conclusion based on facts, not making assumptions.

Answer Types
Test takers should avoid answers that go too far in their value judgment. These answers are often distractors, and can be identified by use of words like *always*, *never*, *only*, and *must*. These absolutes are tough to prove, and likely not to be inferred. The words to look for in the answers to inference questions are *some*, *most*, *can*, and *possibly*, because these are far more likely to indicate an inferred conclusion. Another distractor is an answer that is based on a different subject altogether. This is likely not the answer to an inference question, and can typically be thrown out.

Sample Question
   Congress passed the Older Americans Act (OAA) in 1965 in response to concern by policymakers about a lack of community social services for older persons. The original legislation established authority for grants to States for community planning and social services, research and development projects, and personnel training in the field of aging. The law also established the Administration on Aging (AoA) to administer the newly created grant programs and to serve as the Federal focal point on matters concerning older persons.

   Although older individuals may receive services under many other Federal programs, today the OAA is considered to be the major vehicle for the organization and delivery of social and nutrition services to this group and their caregivers. It authorizes a wide array of service programs through a national network of 56 State agencies on aging, 629 area agencies on aging, nearly 20,000 service providers, 244 Tribal organizations, and 2 Native Hawaiian organizations representing 400 Tribes. The OAA also includes community service employment for low-income older Americans; training, research, and demonstration activities in the field of aging; and vulnerable elder rights protection activities. – Adapted from AOA.gov

1. Based on the above passage, which of the following must be true?
   a. The OAA needs additional funding from the private sector.
   b. Native Hawaiians are always underrepresented in the OAA.
   c. The elderly are in need of protection of their rights.
   d. Nutrition needs of the elderly are severely neglected in this country.

The best answer here is *C*. The author's main idea in this passage is that the OAA was created and exists to provide social services and protect the rights of the elderly. Based on this information, it can be logically inferred that the author believes the elderly need protection of their rights.

Choice *A* is incorrect because the passage mentions that the OAA is funded through grants, and there is no indication of a need for additional funding. It would be an assumption, not an inference, to conclude that more funding is needed from the private sector.

Choice *B* uses an absolute with the use of "never." Use of an absolute could be an indicator of an incorrect answer. While there are only two Native Hawaiian organizations identified as being represented by the OAA in the passage, it states that they represent 400 Tribes. This does not suggest an underrepresentation of this group in the OAA.

Choice *D* requires an assumption, not inference, based on the author's premises. The passage states that the OAA was created in response to a lack of services for the elderly. The OAA has become the biggest organization meeting the nutritional needs of the elderly, so it cannot be inferred that their nutritional needs are being neglected. This answer requires assumption, not inference, based on the author's premises.

Affixes

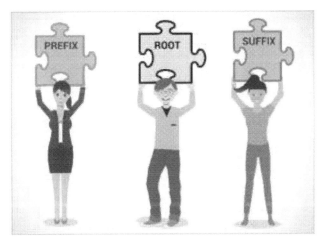

Individual words are constructed from building blocks of meaning. An *affix* is an element that is added to a root or stem word that can change the word's meaning.

For example, the stem word *fix* is a verb meaning *to repair*. When the ending *–able* is added, it becomes the adjective *fixable*, meaning "capable of being repaired." Adding *un–* to the beginning changes the word to *unfixable*, meaning "incapable of being repaired." In this way, affixes attach to the word stem to create a new word and a new meaning. Knowledge of affixes can assist in deciphering the meaning of unfamiliar words.

Affixes are also related to inflection. *Inflection* is the modification of a base word to express a different grammatical or syntactical function. For example, countable nouns such as *car* and *airport* become plural with the addition of *–s* at the end: *cars* and *airports*.

Verb tense is also expressed through inflection. *Regular verbs*—those that follow a standard inflection pattern—can be changed to past tense using the affixes *–ed*, *–d*, or *–ied*, as in *cooked* and *studied*. Verbs can also be modified for continuous tenses by using *–ing*, as in *working* or *exploring*. Thus, affixes are used not only to express meaning but also to reflect a word's grammatical purpose.

A *prefix* is an affix attached to the beginning of a word. The meanings of English prefixes mainly come from Greek and Latin origins. The chart below contains a few of the most commonly used English prefixes.

Prefix	Meaning	Example
a-	Not	amoral, asymptomatic
anti-	Against	antidote, antifreeze
auto-	Self	automobile, automatic
circum-	Around	circumference, circumspect
co-, com-, con-	Together	coworker, companion
contra-	Against	contradict, contrary
de-	negation or reversal	deflate, deodorant
extra-	outside, beyond	extraterrestrial, extracurricular
in-, im-, il-, ir-	Not	impossible, irregular
inter-	Between	international, intervene
intra-	Within	intramural, intranet
mis-	Wrongly	mistake, misunderstand
mono-	One	monolith, monopoly
non-	Not	nonpartisan, nonsense
pre-	Before	preview, prediction
re-	Again	review, renew
semi-	Half	semicircle, semicolon
sub-	Under	subway, submarine
super-	Above	superhuman, superintendent
trans-	across, beyond, through	trans-Siberian, transform
un-	Not	unwelcome, unfriendly

While the addition of a prefix alters the meaning of the base word, the addition of a *suffix* may also affect a word's part of speech. For example, adding a suffix can change the noun *material* into the verb *materialize* and back to a noun again in *materialization*.

Suffix	Part of Speech	Meaning	Example
-able, -ible	adjective	having the ability to	honorable, flexible
-acy, -cy	noun	state or quality	intimacy, dependency
-al, -ical	adjective	having the quality of	historical, tribal
-en	verb	to cause to become	strengthen, embolden
-er, -ier	adjective	comparative	happier, longer
-est, -iest	adjective	superlative	sunniest, hottest
-ess	noun	female	waitress, actress
-ful	adjective	full of, characterized by	beautiful, thankful
-fy, -ify	verb	to cause, to come to be	liquefy, intensify
-ism	noun	doctrine, belief, action	Communism, Buddhism
-ive, -ative, -itive	adjective	having the quality of	creative, innovative
-ize	verb	to convert into, to subject to	Americanize, dramatize
-less	adjective	without, missing	emotionless, hopeless
-ly	adverb	in the manner of	quickly, energetically
-ness	noun	quality or state	goodness, darkness
-ous, -ious, -eous	adjective	having the quality of	spontaneous, pious
-ship	noun	status or condition	partnership, ownership
-tion	noun	action or state	renovation, promotion
-y	adjective	characterized by	smoky, dreamy

Through knowledge of prefixes and suffixes, a student's vocabulary can be instantly expanded with an understanding of *etymology*—the origin of words. This, in turn, can be used to add sentence structure variety to academic writing.

Syntax

Syntax refers to the arrangement of words, phrases, and clauses to form a sentence. Knowledge of syntax can also give insight into a word's meaning. The section above considered several examples using the word *reservation* and applied context clues to determine the word's appropriate meaning in each sentence. Here is an example of how the placement of a word can impact its meaning and grammatical function:

A. The development team has reserved the conference room for today.

B. Her quiet and reserved nature is sometimes misinterpreted as unfriendliness when people first meet her.

In addition to using *reserved* to mean different things, each sentence also uses the word to serve a different grammatical function. In sentence A, *reserved* is part of the verb phrase *has reserved*, indicating the meaning "to set aside for a particular use." In sentence B, *reserved* acts as a modifier within the noun phrase "her quiet and reserved nature." Because the word is being used as an adjective to describe a personality characteristic, it calls up a different definition of the word—"restrained or lacking familiarity with others." As this example shows, the function of a word within the overall sentence structure can allude to its meaning. It is also useful to refer to the earlier chart about suffixes and parts of speech as another clue into what grammatical function a word is serving in a sentence.

The Purpose of Words or Phrases as Used in Context

Knowledge of synonyms and antonyms is crucial for writing and identifying a good paraphrase, and it also helps readers expand their mental vocabulary network. Another useful vocabulary skill is being able to understand meaning in context. A word's context refers to all the other words and information surrounding it, and the context of a word can have an impact on how readers interpret that word's meaning. Of course, many words have more than one definition. For example, consider the meaning of the word *engaged*. The first definition that comes to mind might be "promised to be married," but consider the following sentences:

A. The two armies engaged in a conflict that lasted all night.
B. The three-hour lecture flew by because students were so engaged in the material.
C. The busy executive engaged a new assistant to help with his workload.

As you can see, *engaged* has a variety of other meanings. In these sentences, respectively, it can mean: "battled," "interested or involved," and "appointed or employed." With so many possible definitions, readers may wonder how to decide which one to apply in a given sentence. The appropriate meaning is prioritized based on context. For example, sentence *C* mentions "executive," "assistant," and "workload," so readers can assume that *engaged* has something to do with work—in which case, "appointed or employed" would be the best definition for this context. Context clues can also be found in sentence *A*. Words like "armies" and "conflicts" show that this sentence is about a military situation (and not about marriage or the office), so in this context, *engaged* is closest in meaning to "battled." By using context clues—the surrounding words in the sentence—readers can easily select the most appropriate definition for the word in question.

In addition to helping readers select the best meaning for a word with many definitions, context clues can also help readers when they don't know any meanings for a certain word. Test writers will deliberately ask about vocabulary that test takers are probably unfamiliar with in order to measure their ability to use context to make an educated guess about a word's meaning.

Which of the following is the closest in meaning to the word *loquacious* in the following sentence? The loquacious professor was notorious for always taking too long to finish his lectures.
a. Knowledgeable
b. Enthusiastic
c. Approachable
d. Talkative

Even if the word *loquacious* seems completely new, it is still possible to utilize context to make a good guess about the word's meaning. Grammatically, it is apparent that *loquacious* is an adjective that modifies the noun "professor"—so *loquacious* must be some kind of quality or characteristic. A clue in this sentence is "taking too long to finish his lectures." Readers should then brainstorm qualities that might cause a professor to be late. Perhaps he is "disorganized," "slow," or "talkative"—all words that might still make sense in this sentence. After brainstorming some ideas for the word's definition, take a look at the choices for the question. Choice *D* matches one word from the brainstorming session, and it is a logical choice for this sentence—the professor talks too much, so his lectures run late. In fact, *loquacious* means "talkative" or "wordy."

One way that readers can use context clues is to think of potential replacement words before considering the answer choices given in the question. However, if it is truly a struggle to come up with any possibilities, readers should turn to the answer choices first and try to replace each of them in the sentence to see if the sentence is still logical and retains the same meaning.

Which of the following is the closest in meaning to the word *dogma* in the following sentence? Martin Luther was a revolutionary religious figure because he argued against Catholic dogma and encouraged a new interpretation of Christianity.

    a. Punishments
    b. Doctrines
    c. Leadership
    d. Procedures

Based on context, this sentence has something to do with religious conflict and interpretations of Christian faith. The only word related to religious belief is Choice *B*, *doctrines*, which is in fact the best synonym for *dogma*.

Yet another way to use context clues is to consider clues in the word itself. Most students are probably familiar with prefixes, suffixes, and root words—the building blocks of many English words. A little knowledge goes a long way when it comes to these components of English vocabulary, and they can point readers in the right direction when they need help finding an appropriate definition.

Which of the following is the closest in meaning to the word *antipathy* in the following sentence? A strong antipathy existed between Margaret and her new neighbor, Susan.

    a. Enmity
    b. Resemblance
    c. Relationship
    d. Alliance

In this case, the sentence does not provide much context for the word *antipathy*. However, the word itself gives some useful clues. The prefix *anti-* means "opposite or against," so *antipathy* probably has a negative meaning. Also, if readers already know words like "sympathy" or "empathy," they might guess that the root word "path" is related to emotions. So, *antipathy* must be a feeling *against* something. *Alliance* is a positive connection, *relationship* is too neutral, and *resemblance* means two things are similar to each other. The only word that shows a negative or opposite feeling is Choice *A*, *enmity* (the feeling of being enemies). In this way, even an unfamiliar word contains clues that can indicate its meaning.

The Organization or Structure

Good writing is not merely a random collection of sentences. No matter how well written, sentences must relate and coordinate appropriately to one another. If not, the writing seems random, haphazard, and disorganized. Therefore, good writing must be organized, where each sentence fits a larger context and relates to the sentences around it.

Text Structures
Depending on what the author is attempting to accomplish, certain formats or text structures work better than others. For example, a sequence structure might work for narration but not when identifying similarities and differences between dissimilar concepts. Similarly, a comparison-contrast

structure is not useful for narration. It's the author's job to put the right information in the correct format.

Readers should be familiar with the five main literary structures:

Sequence Structure
Sequence structure, sometimes referred to as the order structure, is when the order of events proceeds in a predictable order. In many cases, this means the text goes through the plot elements: exposition, rising action, climax, falling action, and resolution. Readers are introduced to the characters, setting, and conflict in the *exposition*. In the *rising action*, there's an increase in tension and suspense. The *climax* is the height of tension and the point of no return. Tension decreases during the *falling action*. In the *resolution*, any conflicts presented in the exposition are resolved, and the story concludes. An informative text that is structured sequentially will often go in order from one step to the next.

Problem-Solution
In the problem-solution structure, authors identify a potential problem and suggest a solution. This form of writing is usually divided into two paragraphs and can be found in informational texts. For example, cellphone, cable, and satellite providers use this structure in manuals to help customers troubleshoot or identify problems with services or products.

Comparison-Contrast
When authors want to discuss similarities and differences between separate concepts, they arrange thoughts in a comparison-contrast paragraph structure. Venn diagrams are an effective graphic organizer for comparison-contrast structures, because they feature two overlapping circles that can be used to organize similarities and differences. A comparison-contrast essay organizes one paragraph based on similarities and another based on differences. A comparison-contrast essay can also be arranged with the similarities and differences of individual traits addressed within individual paragraphs. Words such as *however*, *but*, and *nevertheless* help signal a contrast in ideas.

Descriptive
Descriptive writing structure is designed to appeal to the reader's senses. Much like an artist who constructs a painting, good descriptive writing builds an image in the reader's mind by appealing to the five senses: sight, hearing, taste, touch, and smell. However, overly descriptive writing can become tedious; likewise, sparse descriptions can make settings and characters seem flat. Good authors strike a balance by applying descriptions only to facts that are integral to the passage.

Cause and Effect
Passages that use the cause and effect structure are simply asking *why* by demonstrating some type of connection between ideas. Words such as *if*, *since*, *because*, *then*, or *consequently* indicate this relationship. By switching the order of a complex sentence, the writer can rearrange the emphasis on different clauses. Saying *If Sheryl is late, we'll miss the dance* is different from saying *We'll miss the dance if Sheryl is late*. The first example emphasizes Sheryl's tardiness while the other emphasizes missing the dance. Paragraphs can also be arranged in a cause and effect format. Since the format—before and after—is sequential, it is useful when authors wish to discuss the impact of choices. Researchers often apply this paragraph structure to the scientific method.

Transition Words

The writer should act as a guide, showing the reader how all the sentences fit together. Consider this example:

> Seat belts save more lives than any other automobile safety feature. Many studies show that airbags save lives as well. Not all cars have airbags. Many older cars don't. Air bags aren't entirely reliable. Studies show that in 15% of accidents, airbags don't deploy as designed. Seat belt malfunctions are extremely rare.

There's nothing wrong with any of these sentences individually, but together they're disjointed and difficult to follow. The best way for the writer to communicate information smoothly is with transition words. Here are examples of transition words and phrases that tie sentences together, enabling a more natural flow:

- To show causality: as a result, therefore, and consequently
- To compare and contrast: *however, but*, and *on the other hand*
- To introduce examples: *for instance, namely*, and *including*
- To show order of importance: *foremost, primarily, secondly*, and *lastly*

NOTE: This is not a complete list of transitions. There are many more that can be used; however, most fit into these or similar categories. The point is that the words should clearly show the relationship between sentences, supporting information, and the main idea.

Here is an update to the previous example using transition words. These changes make it easier to read and bring clarity to the writer's points:

> Seat belts save more lives than any other automobile safety feature. Many studies show that airbags save lives as well; however, not all cars have airbags. For instance, some older cars don't. Furthermore, air bags aren't entirely reliable. For example, studies show that in 15% of accidents, airbags don't deploy as designed, but, on the other hand, seat belt malfunctions are extremely rare.

Test takers should also be prepared to analyze whether the writer is using the best transition word or phrase for the situation. Take this sentence for example: "As a result, seat belt malfunctions are extremely rare." This sentence doesn't make sense in the context above because the writer is trying to show the contrast between seat belts and airbags, not the causality.

Logical Sequence

Even if the writer includes plenty of information to support his or her point, the writing is only coherent when the information is in a logical order. Logical sequencing is really just common sense, but it's an important writing technique. First, the writer should introduce the main idea, whether for a paragraph, a section, or the entire piece. Then they should present evidence to support the main idea by using transitional language. This shows the reader how the information relates to the main idea and the sentences around it. The writer should then take time to interpret the information, making sure necessary connections are obvious to the reader. Finally, the writer can summarize the information in a closing section.

NOTE: Although most writing follows this pattern, it isn't a set rule. Sometimes writers change the order for effect. For example, the writer can begin with a surprising piece of supporting information to grab the reader's attention, and then transition to the main idea. Thus, if a passage doesn't follow the logical order, test takers should not immediately assume it's wrong. However, most writing usually settles into a logical sequence after a nontraditional beginning.

Introductions and Conclusions

Examining the writer's strategies for introductions and conclusions puts the reader in the right mindset to interpret the rest of the text. Test takers should look for methods the writer might use for introductions such as:

- Stating the main point immediately, followed by outlining how the rest of the piece supports this claim.

- Establishing important, smaller pieces of the main idea first, and then grouping these points into a case for the main idea.

- Opening with a quotation, anecdote, question, seeming paradox, or other piece of interesting information, and then using it to lead to the main point.

- Whatever method the writer chooses, the introduction should make his or her intention clear, establish his or her voice as a credible one, and encourage a person to continue reading.

Conclusions tend to follow a similar pattern. In them, the writer restates his or her main idea a final time, often after summarizing the smaller pieces of that idea. If the introduction uses a quote or anecdote to grab the reader's attention, the conclusion often makes reference to it again. Whatever way the writer chooses to arrange the conclusion, the final restatement of the main idea should be clear and simple for the reader to interpret. Finally, conclusions shouldn't introduce any new information.

Reasoning Within the Text

Integrating Different Components of the Text to Increase Comprehension

Principles that Function Within a Selection

A principle can be defined as a fundamental truth that functions as the foundation of a system of belief, behavior, or reasoning. Expressed another way, a principle is a core truth that cannot be violated. The MCAT examiners write Critical Analysis and Reasoning Skills passages that rely on or express some principle, and the most common principle questions ask test takers to correctly identify the principle expressed in the passage. In addition, some question stems will provide a principle, state that it is true, and ask the test taker to select the answer choice that best describes how the stated principle impacts the passage. The Critical Analysis and Reasoning Skills section also might be composed of two passages, where one passage commonly states the principle, while the other applies it. Principle question stems are typically easy to identify since they will explicitly include the word *principle* or a synonym. Here is an example of a principle question stem:

> The reasoning in the passage most conforms to which of the following principles?

The overwhelming majority of principle questions will list the principles as answer choices, and the test taker should select the principle that best matches the passage.

The MCAT requires test takers to analyze and apply myriad concepts; however, determining a principle's validity will never be a question. If the author asserts the principle that all capitalist economic systems are doomed to fail and asks test takers to identify the principle, then they should select the answer stating that all capitalist systems are doomed to fail. No matter how sensational, the real-world validity of the principle is never in question. By their very definition, principles are outcome determinatives for any situation falling within its universe. Thus, the question that a test taker must always ask is: assuming this principle is true, how does it impact or match the given situation? If the principle is valid, which is assumed in the MCAT, and the specific circumstances fall within the principle's criteria, then the conclusion must adhere to the principle. As a result, answering principle questions is just a matter of matching the passage's specifics with the most appropriate principle.

The first step to interpreting principles is determining whether each principle is broad or narrow. Since everything covered by the principle is true, determining the confines will change how many situations the principle controls. Test takers should pay close attention to limiting language, or lack thereof, in the stated principle. Keywords to consider include: *all, every, any, some, never, none, no, anyone, everyone,* and any other similar words that describe an amount of something. Difference in language will decide whether some action or statement will, could, or could not happen, or be true. In addition, test takers should look for limitations on the group required for the principle to be activated. If the principle's stated limitation excludes some category or requires some characteristic, then it will not apply in situations not covered by the limitation. Consider the difference between the following principles:

- Every American will vote in the upcoming presidential election.
- All Americans interested in politics will vote in the upcoming presidential election.

- Some Americans will vote in the upcoming presidential election.
- No Americans will vote in the upcoming presidential election.

What do these principles say about an individual American? The first principle dictates that the simple fact that the individual is American necessitates that he or she will vote in the upcoming presidential election. As discussed at length above, the test taker must not consider external facts, such as the voting rate being substantially lower than one hundred percent in every American presidential election. This type of principle is outcome determinative for anyone who is an American. If you are an American, then you will vote in the upcoming presidential election. Although the second principle begins with *all*, it includes a limiting requirement, "interested in politics," that must be accounted for in the analysis. It is unclear whether the individual American is interested in politics, and there is no way to find out that fact with the information provided; thus, this principle does not force any conclusion in this situation. The third principle only tells us that some Americans will vote; thus, it is both possible that the individual American will and will not vote, but no outcome is forced. The fourth principle is similar to the first principle since it is outcome determinative. The individual is American; no Americans will vote in the upcoming presidential election; thus, the individual will not be voting. This type of analysis should be used to determine what principle best matches the passage.

Principles can sometimes be converted into *if-then* statements, also known as *conditional statements*, which allow for inferences to be drawn. These inferences provide additional information that is useful for identifying the passage's principle. Before drawing an inference is possible, the principle must be converted into a conditional statement. For example:

> Original: Every American will vote in the upcoming presidential election.
>
> Conversion: If an individual is American, then that individual will vote in the upcoming presidential election.
>
> Representation: A → V (American → Vote)

In this scenario, the knowledge that an individual is an American functions as a sufficient condition, since knowing that fact alone is sufficient to knowing something else—that individual will vote. Voting is referred to as the necessary condition since it necessarily must occur if the sufficient condition is triggered. Conditional statements can also be negated and flipped to reveal a second inference. This is known as the *contrapositive*. The example can be restated as the following:

> Contrapositive: If an individual will not vote in the upcoming presidential election, then that individual is not an American.
>
> Representation: ~~V~~ → ~~A~~ (~~Vote~~ → ~~American~~)

When writing the contrapositive, crossing out the symbol is shorthand for *not*. Depending on the complexity of the principle, as well as the test taker's familiarity with conditional statements, converting the principle might not be feasible in terms of time management. However, if possible, test takers should be cognizant of the effectiveness of conditional statements in evaluating principle questions.

Tricks & Fallacies

Naturally, some of the questions will be more difficult than others. But this also means that answer choices will be intentionally misleading. The following contains logical tricks that may be on the test.

Red Herring

A *red herring* is a logical fallacy in which irrelevant information is introduced to alter the argument's trajectory. Red herrings are the irrelevant information used to fallaciously and slyly divert the argument into an unrelated topic. This fallacy is common in thriller movies or television shows in which the audience is led to believe that a character is the villain or mastermind, while the true villain remains a secret. In terms of the Logical Reasoning section, red herrings will attempt to distract the reader with irrelevant information in either the question or answer choice. A red herring is sometimes referred to as a *straw man*, since this fallacy attacks a different argument than the one presented. Consider the following example of a red herring:

> The government must immediately issue tax cuts to strengthen the economy. A strong middle class is the backbone of a fully functional economy, and tax cuts will increase the discretionary spending necessary to support the middle class. After all, it's extremely important for our society to be open-minded and to limit racial discord.

On its face, the argument looks fine. The conclusion is obvious—the government needs to pass tax cuts to strengthen the economy. This is based on the premise that the cuts will increase discretionary spending, which will strengthen the middle class, and the economy will be stronger. However, the last sentence is a red herring. The argument does not address how a society should be open-minded and avoid racism; it holds no connection with the main thrust of the argument. In this scenario, look out for answer choices that address the red herring rather than the essential argument.

Red herrings will be extremely common in the answer choices. The test makers know that test takers are aware of sound logic and flawed reasoning, but they also know that test takers are working quickly to identify key words and phrases. As a result, the test makers will include many red herrings in the answer choices.

Extreme Language

The test makers commonly write appealing answer choices, but take the language to such an unjustified extreme that it is rendered incorrect. The extreme language usually will take the argument too far.

An example of an argument appealing to the extreme is:

> Weight lifting breaks down muscles and rebuilds them. If one just kept exercising and never stopped, his or her body would deteriorate and eventually fall apart.

This argument is clearly illogical. The author correctly describes what weight lifting does to the body, but then takes the argument to an unjustified extreme. If someone continually lifted weights, his or her body would not deteriorate and fall apart due to the weights breaking down muscle. The weightlifter may eventually die from a heart attack or dehydration, but it would not be because of how weight lifting rebuilds muscle.

Fallacies

A fallacy is a mistaken belief or faulty reasoning, otherwise known as a *logical fallacy*. It is important for readers to recognize logical fallacies because they discredit the author's message. Readers should continuously self-question as they go through a text to identify logical fallacies. Readers cannot simply complacently take information at face value. There are six common types of logical *fallacies:*

1. False analogy
2. Circular reasoning
3. False dichotomy
4. Overgeneralization
5. Slippery slope
6. Hasty generalization

Each of the six logical fallacies are reviewed individually.

False Analogy

A *false analogy* is when the author assumes two objects or events are alike in all aspects despite the fact that they may be vastly different. Authors intend on making unfamiliar objects relatable to convince readers of something. For example, the letters *A* and *E* are both vowels; therefore, *A* = *E*. Readers cannot assume that because *A* and *E* are both vowels that they perform the same function in words or independently. If authors tell readers, *A* = *E*, then that is a false analogy. While this is a simple example, other false analogies may be less obvious.

Circular reasoning

Circular reasoning is when the reasoning is decided based upon the outcome or conclusion and then vice versa. Basically, those who use circular reasoning start out with the argument and then use false logic to try to prove it, and then, in turn, the reasoning supports the conclusion in one big circular pattern. For example, consider the two thoughts, "I don't have time to get organized" and "My disorganization is costing me time." Which is the argument? What is the conclusion? If there is not time to get organized, will more time be spent later trying to find whatever is needed? In turn, if so much time is spent looking for things, there is not time to get organized. The cycle keeps going in an endless series. One problem affects the other; therefore, there is a circular pattern of reasoning.

False dichotomy

A *false dichotomy,* also known as a false dilemma, is when the author tries to make readers believe that there are only two options to choose from when, in fact, there are more. The author creates a false sense of the situation because he or she wants the readers to believe that his or her claim is the most logical choice. If the author does not present the readers with options, then the author is purposefully limiting what readers may believe. In turn, the author hopes that readers will believe that his or her point of view is the most sensible choice. For example, in the statement: *you either love running, or you are lazy*, the fallacy lies in the options of loving to run or being lazy. Even though both statements do not necessarily have to be true, the author tries to make one option seem more appealing than the other.

Overgeneralization

An *overgeneralization* is a logical fallacy that occurs when authors write something so extreme that it cannot be proved or disproved. Words like *all, never, most,* and *few* are commonly used when an overgeneralization is being made. For example,

> All kids are crazy when they eat sugar; therefore, my son will not have a cupcake at the birthday party.

Not *all* kids are crazy when they eat sugar, but the extreme statement can influence the readers' points of view on the subject. Readers need to be wary of overgeneralizations in texts because authors may try to sneak them in to sway the readers' opinions.

Slippery slope

A *slippery slope* is when an author implies that something will inevitably happen as a result of another action. A slippery slope may or may not be true, even though the order of events or gradations may seem logical. For example, in the children's book *If You Give a Mouse a Cookie*, the author goes off on tangents such as "If you give a mouse a cookie, he will ask for some milk. When you give him the milk, he'll probably ask you for a straw." The mouse in the story follows a series of logical events as a result of a previous action. The slippery slope continues on and on throughout the story. Even though the mouse made logical decisions, it very well could have made a different choice, changing the direction of the story.

Hasty generalization

A *hasty generalization* is when the reader comes to a conclusion without reviewing or analyzing all the evidence. It is never a good idea to make a decision without all the information, which is why hasty generalizations are considered fallacies. For example, if two friends go to a hairdresser and give the hairdresser a positive recommendation, that does not necessarily mean that a new client will have the same experience. Two referrals is not quite enough information to form an educated and well-formed conclusion.

Overall, readers should carefully review and analyze authors' arguments to identify logical fallacies and come to sensible conclusions.

Text Evidence

Text evidence is the information readers find in a text or passage that supports the main idea or point(s) in a story. In turn, text evidence can help readers draw conclusions about the text or passage. The information should be taken directly from the text or passage and placed in quotation marks. Text evidence provides readers with information to support ideas about the text so that they do not rely simply on their own thoughts. Details should be precise, descriptive, and factual. Statistics are a great piece of text evidence because they provide readers with exact numbers and not just a generalization. For example, instead of saying "Asia has a larger population than Europe," authors could provide detailed information such as, "In Asia there are over 4 billion people, whereas in Europe there are a little over 750 million." More definitive information provides better evidence to readers to help support their conclusions about texts or passages.

Text Credibility

Credible sources are important when drawing conclusions because readers need to be able to trust what they are reading. Authors should always use credible sources to help gain the trust of their readers. A text is *credible* when it is believable and the author is objective and unbiased. If readers do not trust an author's words, they may simply dismiss the text completely. For example, if an author writes a persuasive essay, he or she is outwardly trying to sway readers' opinions to align with his or her own. Readers may agree or disagree with the author, which may, in turn, lead them to believe that the author is credible or not credible. Also, readers should keep in mind the source of the text. If readers review a journal about astronomy, would a more reliable source be a NASA employee or a medical doctor? Overall, text credibility is important when drawing conclusions, because readers want reliable sources that support the decisions they have made about the author's ideas.

Counterarguments

If an author presents a differing opinion or a counterargument in order to refute it, the reader should consider how and why this information is being presented. It is meant to strengthen the original argument and shouldn't be confused with the author's intended conclusion, but it should also be considered in the reader's final evaluation.

Authors can also use bias if they ignore the opposing viewpoint or present their side in an unbalanced way. A strong argument considers the opposition and finds a way to refute it. Critical readers should look for an unfair or one-sided presentation of the argument and be skeptical, as a bias may be present. Even if this bias is unintentional, if it exists in the writing, the reader should be wary of the validity of the argument. Readers should also look for the use of stereotypes, which refer to specific groups. Stereotypes are often negative connotations about a person or place, and should always be avoided. When a critical reader finds stereotypes in a piece of writing, they should be critical of the argument, and consider the validity of anything the author presents. Stereotypes reveal a flaw in the writer's thinking and may suggest a lack of knowledge or understanding about the subject.

Opinions, Facts, and Fallacies

As mentioned previously, authors write with a purpose. They adjust their writing for an intended audience. It is the readers' responsibility to comprehend the writing style or purpose of the author. When readers understand a writer's purpose, they can then form their own thoughts about the text(s) regardless of whether their thoughts are the same as or different from the author's. The following section will examine different writing tactics that authors use, such as facts versus opinions, bias and stereotypes, appealing to the readers' emotions, and fallacies (including false analogies, circular reasoning, false dichotomy, and overgeneralization).

Facts Versus Opinions

Readers need to be aware of the writer's purpose to help discern facts and opinions within texts. A *fact* is a piece of information that is true. It can either prove or disprove claims or arguments presented in texts. Facts cannot be changed or altered. For example, the statement: *Abraham Lincoln was assassinated on April 15, 1865*, is a fact. The date and related events cannot be altered.

Authors not only present facts in their writing to support or disprove their claim(s), but they may also express their opinions. Authors may use factsto support their own opinions, especially in a persuasive text; however, that does not make their opinions facts. An *opinion* is a belief or view formed about something that is not necessarily based on the truth. Opinions often express authors' personal feelings about a subject and use words like *believe, think,* or *feel.* For example, the statement: *Abraham Lincoln was the best president who has ever lived*, expresses the writer's opinion. Not all writers or readers agree or disagree with the statement. Therefore, the statement can be altered or adjusted to express opposing or supporting beliefs, such as "Abraham Lincoln was the worst president who has ever lived" or "I also think Abraham Lincoln was a great president."

When authors include facts and opinions in their writing, readers may be less influenced by the text(s). Readers need to be conscious of the distinction between facts and opinions while going through texts. Not only should the intended audience be vigilant in following authors' thoughts versus valid information, readers need to check the source of the facts presented. Facts should have reliable sources derived from credible outlets like almanacs, encyclopedias, medical journals, and so on.

Bias and Stereotypes

Not only can authors state facts or opinions in their writing, they sometimes intentionally or unintentionally show bias or portray a stereotype. A *bias* is when someone demonstrates a prejudice in favor of or against something or someone in an unfair manner. When an author is biased in his or her writing, readers should be skeptical despite the fact that the author's bias may be correct. For example, two athletes competed for the same position. One athlete is related to the coach and is a mediocre athlete, while the other player excels and deserves the position. The coach chose the less talented player who is related to him for the position. This is a biased decision because it favors someone in an unfair way.

Similar to a bias, a *stereotype* shows favoritism or opposition but toward a specific group or place. Stereotypes create an oversimplified or overgeneralized idea about a certain group, person, or place. For example,

> Women are horrible drivers.

This statement basically labels *all* women as horrible drivers. While there may be some terrible female drivers, the stereotype implies that *all* women are bad drivers when, in fact, not *all* women are. While many readers are aware of several vile ethnic, religious, and cultural stereotypes, audiences should be cautious of authors' flawed assumptions because they can be less obvious than the despicable examples that are unfortunately pervasive in society.

Synthesis

Synthesis in reading involves the ability to fully comprehend text passages, and then going further by making new connections to see things in a new or different way. It involves a full thought process and requires readers to change the way they think about what they read. The MCAT will require a test taker to integrate new information that he or she already knows, and demonstrate an ability to express new thoughts.

Synthesis goes further than summary. When summarizing, a reader collects all of the information an author presents in a text passage, and restates it in an effective manner. Synthesis requires that the test taker not only summarize reading material, but be able to express new ideas based on the author's message. It is a full culmination of all reading comprehension strategies. It will require the test taker to order, recount, summarize, and recreate information into a whole new idea.

In utilizing synthesis, a reader must be able to form mental images about what they read, recall any background information they have about the topic, ask critical questions about the material, determine the importance of points an author makes, make inferences based on the reading, and finally be able to form new ideas based on all of the above skills. Synthesis requires the reader to make connections, visualize concepts, determine their importance, ask questions, make inferences, then fully synthesize all of this information into new thought.

Making Connections in Reading

There are three helpful thinking strategies to keep in mind when attempting to synthesize text passages:

- Think about how the content of a passage relates to life experience;
- Think about how the content of a passage relates to other text and;
- Think about how the content of a passage relates to the world in general.

When reading a given passage, the test taker should actively think about how the content relates to their life experience. While the author's message may express an opinion different from what the reader believes, or express ideas with which the reader is unfamiliar, a good reader will try to relate any of the author's details to their own familiar ground. A reader should use context clues to understand unfamiliar terminology, and recognize familiar information they have encountered in prior experience. Bringing prior life experience and knowledge to the test-taking situation is helpful in making connections. The ability to relate an unfamiliar idea to something the reader already knows is critical in understanding unique and new ideas. When trying to make connections while reading, keep the following questions in mind:

- How does this feel familiar in personal experience?
- How is this similar to or different from other reading?
- How is this familiar in the real world?
- How does this relate to the world in general?

A reader should ask themself these questions during the act of reading in order to actively make connections to past and present experiences. Utilizing the ability to make connections is an important step in achieving synthesis.

Identifying Reading Strategies

A *reading strategy* is the way a reader interacts with text in order to understand its meaning. It is a skill set that a reader brings to the reading. It employs a reader's ability to use prior knowledge when addressing literature and utilizes a set of methods in order to analyze text. A reading strategy is not simply tackling a text passage as it appears. It involves a more complex system of planning and thought during the reading experience. Current research indicates readers who utilize strategies and a variety of critical reading skills are better thinkers who glean more interpretive information from their reading. Consequently, they are more successful in their overall comprehension.

Pre-Reading Strategies

Pre-reading strategies are important, yet often overlooked. Non-critical readers will often begin reading without taking the time to review factors that will help them understand the text. Skipping pre-reading strategies may result in a reader having to re-address a text passage more times than is necessary. Some pre-reading strategies include the following:

- Previewing the text for clues
- Skimming the text for content
- Scanning for unfamiliar words in context
- Formulating questions on sight

- Making predictions
- Recognizing needed prior knowledge

Before reading a text passage, a reader can enhance his or her ability to comprehend material by *previewing the text for clues*. This may mean making careful note of any titles, headings, graphics, notes, introductions, important summaries, and conclusions. It can involve a reader making physical notes regarding these elements or highlighting anything he or she thinks is important before reading. Often, a reader will be able to gain information just from these elements alone. Of course, close reading is required in order to fill in the details. A reader needs to be able to ask what he or she is reading about and what a passage is trying to say. The answers to these general questions can often be answered in previewing the text itself.

It's helpful to use pre-reading clues to determine the main idea and organization. First, any titles, sub-headings, chapter headings should be read, and the test taker should make note of the author's credentials if any are listed. It's important to deduce what these clues may indicate as it pertains to the focus of the text and how it's organized.

During pre-reading, readers should also take special note of how text features contribute to the central idea or thesis of the passage. Is there an index? Is there a glossary? What headings, footnotes, or other visuals are included and how do they relate to the details within the passage? Again, this is where any pre-reading notes come in handy, since a test taker should be able to relate supporting details to these textual features.

Next, a reader should *skim* the text for general ideas and content. This technique does not involve close reading; rather, it involves looking for important words within the passage itself. These words may have something to do with the author's theme. They may have to do with structure—for example, words such as *first, next, therefore*, and *last*. Skimming helps a reader understand the overall structure of a passage and, in turn, this helps him or her understand the author's theme or message.

From there, a reader should quickly *scan* the text for any unfamiliar words. When reading a print text, highlighting these words or making other marginal notation is helpful when going back to read text critically. A reader should look at the words surrounding any unfamiliar ones to see what contextual clues unfamiliar words carry. Being able to define unfamiliar terms through contextual meaning is a critical skill in reading comprehension.

A reader should also *formulate any questions* he or she might have before conducting close reading. Questions such as "What is the author trying to tell me?" or "Is the author trying to persuade my thinking?" are important to a reader's ability to engage critically with the text. Questions will focus a reader's attention on what is important in terms of idea and what is supporting detail.

Along with formulating questions, it is helpful to make predictions of what the answers to these questions and others will be. *Making predictions* involves using information from the text and personal experiences to make a thoughtful guess as to what will happen in the story and what outcomes can be expected.

Last, a reader should recognize that author's assume readers bring a *prior knowledge* set to the reading experience. Not all readers have the same experience, but authors seek to communicate with their readers. In turn, readers should strive to interact with the author of a particular passage by asking themselves what the passage demands they know during reading. This is also known as making a text-to-self connection. If a passage is informational in nature, a reader should ask "What do I know about this topic from other experiences I've had or other works I've read?" If a reader can relate to the content, he or she will better understand it.

All of the above pre-reading strategies will help the reader prepare for a closer reading experience. They will engage a reader in active interaction with the text by helping to focus the reader's full attention on the details that he or she will encounter during the next round or two of critical, closer reading.

Strategies During Reading

After pre-reading, a test taker can employ a variety of other reading strategies while conducting one or more closer readings. These strategies include the following:

- Clarifying during a close read
- Questioning during a close read
- Organizing the main ideas and supporting details
- Summarizing the text effectively

A reader needs to be able to *clarify* what he or she is reading. This strategy demands a reader think about how and what he or she is reading. This thinking should occur during and after the act of reading. For example, a reader may encounter one or more unfamiliar ideas during reading, then be asked to apply thoughts about those unfamiliar concepts after reading when answering test questions.

Questioning during a critical read is closely related to clarifying. A reader must be able to ask questions in general about what he or she is reading and questions regarding the author's supporting ideas. Questioning also involves a reader's ability to self-question. When closely reading a passage, it's not enough to simply try and understand the author. A reader must consider critical thinking questions to ensure he or she is comprehending intent. It's advisable, when conducting a close read, to write out margin notes and questions during the experience. These questions can be addressed later in the thinking process after reading and during the phase where a reader addresses the test questions. A reader who is successful in reading comprehension will iteratively question what he or she reads, search text for clarification, then answer any questions that arise.

A reader should *organize* main ideas and supporting details cognitively as he or she reads, as it will help the reader understand the larger structure at work. The use of quick annotations or marks to indicate what the main idea is and how the details function to support it can be helpful. Understanding the structure of a text passage is sometimes critical to answering questions about an author's approach, theme, messages, and supporting detail. This strategy is most effective when reading informational or nonfiction text. Texts that try to convince readers of a particular idea, that present a theory, or that try to explain difficult concepts are easier to understand when a reader can identify the overarching structure at work.

Post-Reading Strategies

After completing a text, a reader should be able to *summarize* the author's theme and supporting details in order to fully understand the passage. Being able to effectively restate the author's message, sub-themes, and pertinent, supporting ideas will help a reader gain an advantage when addressing standardized test questions.

A reader should also evaluate the strength of the predictions that were made in the pre-reading stage. Using textual evidence, predictions should be compared to the actual events in the story to see if the two were similar or not. Employing all of these strategies will lead to fuller, more insightful reading comprehension.

Reasoning Beyond the Text

Applying Ideas from the Passage to New Contexts

The Application of Information in the Selection to a New Context

A natural extension of being able to make an inference from a given set of information is also being able to apply that information to a new context. This is especially useful in nonfiction or informative writing. Considering the facts and details presented in the text, readers should consider how the same information might be relevant in a different situation. The following is an example of applying an inferential conclusion to a different context:

> Often, individuals behave differently in large groups than they do as individuals. One example of this is the psychological phenomenon known as the bystander effect. According to the bystander effect, the more people who witness an accident or crime occur, the less likely each individual bystander is to respond or offer assistance to the victim. A classic example of this is the murder of Kitty Genovese in New York City in the 1960s. Although there were over thirty witnesses to her killing by a stabber, none of them intervened to help Kitty or contacted the police.

Considering the phenomenon of the bystander effect, what would probably happen if somebody tripped on the stairs in a crowded subway station?
- a. Everybody would stop to help the person who tripped.
- b. Bystanders would point and laugh at the person who tripped.
- c. Someone would call the police after walking away from the station.
- d. Few, if any, bystanders would aid the person who tripped.

This question asks readers to apply the information they learned from the passage, which is an informative paragraph about the bystander effect. According to the passage, this is a concept in psychology that describes the way people in groups respond to an accident—the more people that are present, the less likely any one person is to intervene. While the passage illustrates this effect with the example of a woman's murder, the question asks readers to apply it to a different context—in this case, someone falling down the stairs in front of many subway passengers. Although this specific situation is not discussed in the passage, readers should be able to apply the general concepts described in the paragraph. The definition of the bystander effect includes any instance of an accident or crime in front of a large group of people. The question asks about a situation that falls within the same definition, so the general concept should still hold true: amid a large crowd, few individuals are likely to actually respond to an accident. In this case, answer Choice *D* is the best response.

Analogies to Claims or Arguments in the Selection

Analogous questions challenge test takers' understanding of the passage by asking questions involving the recognition of structurally similar arguments. Test takers often struggle with analogies to claims within a Critical Analysis and Reasoning Skills passage for two reasons. First, analogies inherently test abstract reasoning. The questions ask test takers to draw comparisons between situations that appear entirely unrelated on the surface. Emphasis is placed on logical structure rather than substantive content. For this reason, analogies to claims in the Critical Analysis and Reasoning Skills section are most similar to the parallel reasoning questions that appear in the logical reasoning section. Second, these questions take up a disproportionate amount of finite time relative to other question types.

Due to the abstract nature of these analogy questions, all of the answer choices must be given special scrutiny. It will likely be more difficult to immediately eliminate a choice, since every choice will form its own claim or element. Therefore, test takers must break down each answer choice into its corresponding elements and then compare those elements with the argument or claim from the passage. In addition, the smallest detail will often separate the correct answer from the next best option.

With that said, analogies to claims are not to be feared. Although admittedly cumbersome, they only require completing and repeating one of the most tested concepts on the MCAT—identifying conclusions and determining how premises operate to support those conclusions. The question stem will provide a quote or direct test takers to a set of lines from the passage. Sometimes the quote or line reference will isolate a single claim or argument from the passage, while other times the required interpretation will rely on the passage's broader context. This skill requires using abstract reasoning to draw analogies between situations, and the strongest analogy will typically prevail.

Analogies to claims questions will be easy to identify since *analogous* will almost always appear directly in the question stem. In less common instances, the question stem might include some derivation of application or ask what scenario is *most similar* to the logic deployed in the passage. Here is an example of an analogous question stem:

> Given Friedman's economic theory, as expressed between lines 32 and 45 in the passage, which one of the following is most analogous to the role monetary policy plays in his theory?

When initially reading through the passage, test takers need to pay close attention to differing theories, arguments, or claims, especially from competing sources. For example, a passage about economics might include arguments from two or more economists. In this scenario, the analogous question will always identify which of the competing arguments to analogize. Test takers should never stray from the constraints provided in the question stem. If the economics passage includes arguments from John Maynard Keynes, Milton Friedman, and Karl Marx, but the question only asks how Friedman's theory applies to different scenarios, only focus on the portion of the passage devoted to Friedman. For the purposes of this question, the theories of Keynes and Marx are irrelevant.

The abstract reasoning behind analogous questions forces test takers to compare the logical structure of claims and arguments. The MCAT often includes answer choices that closely mirror the substance of the passage, rather than its structure. Test takers must be careful not to fall for this trick—whether the passage and answer choice discuss the same substantive topic is irrelevant. As a result, test takers should be extremely cautious of answer choices that use similar language or cover identical topics as the claim in the passage. In fact, these type of similar substance answers are usually incorrect, functioning as a red herring to catch the less astute test takers who fail to analyze the structure.

The table below contains some general frameworks that MCAT examiners use to analogize between the passage and answer choices. These are not an exhaustive list of analogous situations included in the

Critical Analysis and Reasoning Skills section; however, reviewing these examples provides a framework for thinking about patterns in analogous questions.

General Structure	Example of an Analogy
Cause and effect	A scientist meticulously attempts a variety of methods and ultimately cures a deadly disease. A student reads her textbook, watches class lectures, and listens to an audio recording from a panel of experts, and she achieves the highest grade in her class.
Part and whole (subset)	All whales are mammals but not all mammals are whales. All prosecutors are lawyers but not all lawyers are prosecutors.
Unintended consequence	A town passes legislation outlawing the hunting of deer to increase their population, but the exploding deer population eats all of the vegetation, and their population decreases. An airline invests in a new silent plane to attract more customers, but their business decreases as customers become irritated with the noise from the bathroom and side conversations that had previously been blocked out by the engine noise.
Confusing causation (especially with correlation)	Ice cream sales rise at the same time as the murder rate similarly increases, but the actual cause of both is more people outside during the summer. A textbook company doubles its sales at the same time the company moves its headquarters to a more prestigious location, but the actual cause of both is an increase in capital investment.
Performance relative to a defined standard	A teenager loses his driver's license after amassing too many points as a result of accidents and speeding tickets. A doctor loses his medical license after a series of patients win medical malpractice actions against him.

To answer analogous questions, the test taker should first reread the passage's discussion of the quote or lines referenced by the question stem. Next, the test taker should generally summarize the structure of the presented claim or argument. For example, many analogous questions ask what logical error the author committed, so the summary would be a short description of that error. This summary should be a slightly more detailed version of what appears in the chart's left column. Lastly, the test taker should make similar summaries for each answer choice, and then the closest match will be the correct answer.

Introducing New Factors, Information, or Conditions to Ideas from the Passage

Critical Analysis and Reasoning Skills question stems will occasionally supplement the passage with new information in the answer choices. The new information will typically impact the conclusion of the entire passage or a supporting claim. The correct answer in a new information question will always do more than merely relate to the same substantive topic as the claim or argument in the passage; the new information will have a direct impact on the claim's plausibility or likelihood. Fortunately, new information questions are essentially strengthening or weakening questions, and the question stem will explicitly specify which of the two is being asked. Here is an example of a weakening question stem:

> Which of the following, if true, would most undermine the author's claim that *Infinite Jest* is the most rewarding book to read?

Here is an example of a strengthening question:

> Which of the following, if true, best supports the author's contention that capitalism is the most effective economic system?

Test takers should notice that the question stem includes the caveat "if true." All new information questions will include such a caveat, so the plausibility or validity of the new information should never be questioned based on real-world knowledge. The new information will likely involve an unaccounted-for fact, expert opinion, recent discovery, or some other substantive statement related to the passage. The next table includes the most common synonyms for *strengthen* or *weaken* to help identify new information questions.

Strengthen	Weaken
Support	Undermine
Fortify	Challenge
Buttress	Diminish
Reinforce	Impair
Fortify	Erode
Bolster	Call into question
Underpin	Lessen
Augment	Undercut
Supplement	Damage

The easiest type of new information question will simply ask which of the following statements weakens or strengthens the claim or argument. If the question stem does not include a modifier, such as *best* or *most*, then only one of the answer choices will weaken or strengthen the claim; it would be impossible for more than one answer choice to strengthen or weaken the claim in such a situation. This makes the question much more approachable, since only one answer choice will impact the argument in the right direction.

When the question does include the *best* or *most* modifier, then multiple answer choices will provide new information that impact the claim in the right direction. In this scenario, the test taker should immediately eliminate any answer choice that does the opposite. For example, if the question asks what best supports a claim, then test takers can eliminate any answer choice that weakens it. In addition, any answer choice that is neutral or irrelevant can be eliminated. Of the remaining answer choices, test takers should select the answer choice that is most relevant to the claim, which usually presents itself by directly addressing the conclusion or an important premise. Similarly, new information questions will occasionally come in the *except* variety. These questions are actually quite similar to the simple weaken or strengthen question, since there will only be one answer choice moving in the right direction. However, test takers should always make sure to read the question stem carefully, or else the question will be impossible to answer correctly.

Test takers often fret over new information questions, believing that the new information will completely fortify or totally deconstruct the argument. Although such extreme scenarios would actually be easier to answer, the correct answer will just make the argument more likely or less likely to be plausible. As with most of the other questions in the Critical Analysis and Reasoning Skills section, identifying conclusions and evaluating premises is by far the most important skill. The correct answers will almost always impact the conclusion by altering the premises.

For strengthen questions, test takers should review the claim or argument in the context of the passage and evaluate its logical strength. Where could the argument be improved? If the weakness is glaring, then the correct answer should be clear amongst the options. The test taker should look out for any new information that validates a prediction or proves a generalization mentioned in the passage. Another possible way to strengthen an argument occurs when the new information provides support for a previously unjustified assumption. In addition, answers to strengthen questions will sometimes come in the form of principles, as discussed above. In these instances, the principle will provide some generalization that impacts a specific statement from the passage. For example, the passage might rely on a supporting claim without any justification, and the principle will strengthen the argument by stating that the claim is always true under those circumstances.

One of the most common answers to strengthen questions is an answer choice that offers new information that will impact the claim by providing a missing link between premises. The original claim or argument might not have connected these two premises, or the new information might strengthen the bridge between premises and the conclusion. Strengthening connections between premises is common when the relevant argument or claim does not immediately appear to be weak or lacking in some way. In the case of already strong arguments, another common correct answer will rule out possible alternatives. For example, the premises might all be airtight, but they collectively lead to two equally plausible conclusions. In this case, the correct answer will rule out the alternative conclusion, and therefore strengthen the conclusion actually included in the claim or argument.

Similarly, in weaken questions, the correct answer will make the argument less plausible by showing that the premises do not necessarily lead to the stated conclusion. This occurs when an important premise is invalidated or eliminated in some way. Special attention should be paid to any premises, suppositions, or statements that rely on some fact being true. Test takers should also pay special attention to how the premises relate to each other in support of the conclusion. Does one premise connect multiple other premises to the argument? If so, then this is the type of premise that is often invalidated by the new information, and the argument will completely fall apart. The more premises that fall off from supporting the conclusion, the weaker the argument. In addition, any new information that invalidates an important prediction or disproves a relied upon generalization will often be the correct answer. Arguments or claims can also be weakened if the new information creates a scenario where an equally plausible alternative conclusion can be drawn. Furthermore, it is possible to weaken arguments by attacking a relied upon assumption.

Practice Questions

Questions 1-6 are based on the following passage:

Dana Gioia argues in his article that poetry is dying, now little more than a limited art form confined to academic and college settings. Of course, poetry remains healthy in the academic setting, but the idea of poetry being limited to this academic subculture is a stretch. New technology and social networking alone have contributed to poets and other writers' work being shared across the world. YouTube has emerged to be a major asset to poets, allowing live performances to be streamed to billions of users. Even now, poetry continues to grow and voice topics that are relevant to the culture of our time. Poetry is not in the spotlight as it may have been in earlier times, but it's still a relevant art form that continues to expand in scope and appeal.

Furthermore, Gioia's argument does not account for live performances of poetry. Not everyone has taken a poetry class or enrolled in university—but most everyone is online. The Internet is a perfect launching point to get all creative work out there. An example of this was the performance of Buddy Wakefield's *Hurling Crowbirds at Mockingbars*. Wakefield is a well-known poet who has published several collections of contemporary poetry. One of my favorite works by Wakefield is *Crowbirds*, specifically his performance at New York University in 2009. Although his reading was a campus event, views of his performance online number in the thousands. His poetry attracted people outside of the university setting.

Naturally, the poem's popularity can be attributed both to Wakefield's performance and the quality of his writing. *Crowbirds* touches on themes of core human concepts such as faith, personal loss, and growth. These are not ideas that only poets or students of literature understand, but all human beings: "You acted like I was hurling crowbirds at mockingbars / and abandoned me for not making sense. / Evidently, I don't experience things as rationally as you do" (Wakefield 15-17). Wakefield weaves together a complex description of the perplexed and hurt emotions of the speaker undergoing a separation from a romantic interest. The line "You acted like I was hurling crowbirds at mockingbars" conjures up an image of someone confused, seemingly out of their mind . . . or in the case of the speaker, passionately trying to grasp at a relationship that is fading. The speaker is looking back and finding the words that described how he wasn't making sense. This poem is particularly human and gripping in its message, but the entire effect of the poem is enhanced through the physical performance.

At its core, poetry is about addressing issues/ideas in the world. Part of this is also addressing the perspectives that are exiguously considered. Although the platform may look different, poetry continues to have a steady audience due to the emotional connection the poet shares with the audience.

1. Which one of the following best explains how the passage is organized?
   a. The author begins with a long definition of the main topic, and then proceeds to prove how that definition has changed over the course of modernity.
   b. The author presents a puzzling phenomenon and uses the rest of the passage to showcase personal experiences in order to explain it.
   c. The author contrasts two different viewpoints, then builds a case showing preference for one over the other.
   d. The passage is an analysis of another theory in which the author has no stake in.

2. The author of the passage would likely agree most with which of the following?
   a. Buddy Wakefield is a genius and is considered at the forefront of modern poetry.
   b. Poetry is not irrelevant; it is an art form that adapts to the changing time while containing its core elements.
   c. Spoken word is the zenith of poetic forms and the premier style of poetry in this decade.
   d. Poetry is on the verge of vanishing from our cultural consciousness.

3. Which one of the following words, if substituted for the word *exiguously* in the last paragraph, would LEAST change the meaning of the sentence?
   a. Indolently
   b. Inaudibly
   c. Interminably
   d. Infrequently

4. Which of the following is most closely analogous to the author's opinion of Buddy Wakefield's performance in relation to modern poetry?
   a. Someone's refusal to accept that the Higgs Boson will validate the Standard Model.
   b. An individual's belief that soccer will lose popularity within the next fifty years.
   c. A professor's opinion that poetry contains the language of the heart, while fiction contains the language of the mind.
   d. A student's insistence that psychoanalysis is a subset of modern psychology.

5. What is the primary purpose of the passage?
   a. To educate readers on the development of poetry and describe the historical implications of poetry in media.
   b. To disprove Dana Gioia's stance that poetry is becoming irrelevant and is only appreciated in academia.
   c. To inform readers of the brilliance of Buddy Wakefield and to introduce them to other poets that have influence in contemporary poetry.
   d. To prove that Gioia's article does have some truth to it and to shed light on its relevance to modern poetry.

6. What is the author's main reason for including the quote in the passage?
   a. The quote opens up opportunity to disprove Gioia's views.
   b. To demonstrate that people are still writing poetry even if the medium has changed in current times.
   c. To prove that poets still have an audience to write for even if the audience looks different than it did centuries ago.
   d. The quote illustrates the complex themes poets continue to address, which still draws listeners and appreciation.

In the quest to understand existence, modern philosophers must question if humans can fully comprehend the world. Classical western approaches to philosophy tend to hold that one can understand something, be it an event or object, by standing outside of the phenomena and observing it. It is then by unbiased observation that one can grasp the details of the world. This seems to hold true for many things. Scientists conduct experiments and record their findings, and thus many natural phenomena become comprehendible. However, several of these observations were possible because humans used tools in order to make these discoveries.

This may seem like an extraneous matter. After all, people invented things like microscopes and telescopes in order to enhance their capacity to view cells or the movement of stars. While humans are still capable of seeing things, the question remains if human beings have the capacity to fully observe and see the world in order to understand it. It would not be an impossible stretch to argue that what humans see through a microscope is not the exact thing itself, but a human interpretation of it.

This would seem to be the case in the "Business of the Holes" experiment conducted by Richard Feynman. To study the way electrons behave, Feynman set up a barrier with two holes and a plate. The plate was there to indicate how many times the electrons would pass through the hole(s). Rather than casually observe the electrons acting under normal circumstances, Feynman discovered that electrons behave in two totally different ways depending on whether or not they are observed. The electrons that were observed had passed through either one of the holes or were caught on the plate as particles. However, electrons that weren't observed acted as waves instead of particles and passed through both holes. This indicated that electrons have a dual nature. Electrons seen by the human eye act like particles, while unseen electrons act like waves of energy.

This dual nature of the electrons presents a conundrum. While humans now have a better understanding of electrons, the fact remains that people cannot entirely perceive how electrons behave without the use of instruments. We can only observe one of the mentioned behaviors, which only provides a partial understanding of the entire function of electrons. Therefore, we're forced to ask ourselves whether the world we observe is objective or if it is subjectively perceived by humans. Or, an alternative question: can man understand the world only through machines that will allow them to observe natural phenomena?

Both questions humble man's capacity to grasp the world. However, those ideas don't consider that many phenomena have been proven by human beings without the use of machines, such as the discovery of gravity. Like all philosophical questions, whether man's reason and observation alone can understand the universe can be approached from many angles.

7. The word *extraneous* in paragraph two can be best interpreted as referring to which one of the following?
    a. Indispensable
    b. Bewildering
    c. Superfluous
    d. Exuberant

8. What is the author's motivation for writing the passage?
    a. To bring to light an alternative view on human perception by examining the role of technology in human understanding.
    b. To educate the reader on the latest astroparticle physics discovery and offer terms that may be unfamiliar to the reader.
    c. To argue that humans are totally blind to the realities of the world by presenting an experiment that proves that electrons are not what they seem on the surface.
    d. To reflect on opposing views of human understanding.

9. Which of the following most closely resembles the way in which paragraph four is structured?
    a. It offers one solution, questions the solution, and then ends with an alternative solution.
    b. It presents an inquiry, explains the details of that inquiry, and then offers a solution.
    c. It presents a problem, explains the details of that problem, and then ends with more inquiry.
    d. It gives a definition, offers an explanation, and then ends with an inquiry.

10. For the classical approach to understanding to hold true, which of the following must be required?
    a. A telescope
    b. A recording device
    c. Multiple witnesses present
    d. The person observing must be unbiased

11. Which best describes how the electrons in the experiment behaved like waves?
    a. The electrons moved up and down like actual waves.
    b. The electrons passed through both holes and then onto the plate.
    c. The electrons converted to photons upon touching the plate.
    d. Electrons were seen passing through one hole or the other.

12. The author mentions "gravity" in the last paragraph in order to do what?
    a. To show that different natural phenomena test man's ability to grasp the world.
    b. To prove that since man has not measured it with the use of tools or machines, humans cannot know the true nature of gravity.
    c. To demonstrate an example of natural phenomena humans discovered and understand without the use of tools or machines.
    d. To show an alternative solution to the nature of electrons that humans have not thought of yet.

13. Which situation best parallels the revelation of the dual nature of electrons discovered in Feynman's experiment?

    a. A man is born color-blind and grows up observing everything in lighter or darker shades. With the invention of special goggles he puts on, he discovers that there are other colors in addition to different shades.

    b. The coelacanth was thought to be extinct, but a live specimen was just recently discovered. There are now two living species of coelacanth known to man, and both are believed to be endangered.

    c. In the Middle Ages, blacksmiths added carbon to iron, thus inventing steel. The consequences of this important discovery would have its biggest effects during the industrial revolution.

    d. In order to better examine and treat broken bones, the x-ray machine was invented and put to use in hospitals and medical centers.

14. Which statement about technology would the author likely disagree with?

    a. Technology can help expand the field of human vision.

    b. Technology renders human observation irrelevant.

    c. Developing tools used in observation and research indicates growing understanding of our world itself.

    d. Studying certain phenomena necessitates the use of tools and machines.

Questions 15-19 are based on the following passage:

The Middle Ages were a time of great superstition and theological debate. Many beliefs were developed and practiced, while some died out or were listed as heresy. Boethianism is a Medieval theological philosophy that attributes sin to gratification and righteousness with virtue and God's providence. Boethianism holds that sin, greed, and corruption are means to attain temporary pleasure, but that they inherently harm the person's soul as well as other human beings.

In *The Canterbury Tales,* we observe more instances of bad actions punished than goodness being rewarded. This would appear to be some reflection of Boethianism. In the "Pardoner's Tale," all three thieves wind up dead, which is a result of their desire for wealth. Each wrong doer pays with their life, and they are unable to enjoy the wealth they worked to steal. Within his tales, Chaucer gives reprieve to people undergoing struggle, but also interweaves stories of contemptible individuals being cosmically punished for their wickedness. The thieves idolize physical wealth, which leads to their downfall. This same theme and ideological principle of Boethianism is repeated in the "Friar's Tale," whose summoner character attempts to gain further wealth by partnering with a demon. The summoner's refusal to repent for his avarice and corruption leads to the demon dragging his soul to Hell. Again, we see the theme of the individual who puts faith and morality aside in favor for a physical prize. The result, of course, is that the summoner loses everything.

The examples of the righteous being rewarded tend to appear in a spiritual context within the *Canterbury Tales*. However, there are a few instances where we see goodness resulting in physical reward. In the Prioress' Tale, we see corporal punishment for barbarism *and* a reward for goodness. The Jews are punished for their murder of the child, giving a sense of law and order (though racist) to the plot. While the boy does die, he is granted a lasting reward by being able to sing even after his death, a miracle that marks that the murdered youth led a pure life. Here, the miracle represents eternal favor with God.

Again, we see the theological philosophy of Boethianism in Chaucer's *The Canterbury Tales* through acts of sin and righteousness and the consequences that follow. When pleasures of the world are sought instead of God's favor, we see characters being punished in tragic ways. However, the absence of worldly lust has its own set of consequences for the characters seeking to obtain God's favor.

15. What would be a potential reward for living a good life, as described in Boethianism?
    a. A long life sustained by the good deeds one has done over a lifetime
    b. Wealth and fertility for oneself and the extension of one's family line
    c. Vengeance for those who have been persecuted by others who have a capacity for committing wrongdoing
    d. God's divine favor for one's righteousness

16. What might be the main reason why the author chose to discuss Boethianism through examining The Canterbury Tales?
    a. *The Canterbury Tales* is a well-known text.
    b. *The Canterbury Tales* is the only known fictional text that contains use of Boethianism.
    c. *The Canterbury Tales* presents a manuscript written in the medieval period that can help illustrate Boethianism through stories and show how people of the time might have responded to the idea.
    d. Within each individual tale in *The Canterbury Tales*, the reader can read about different levels of Boethianism and how each level leads to greater enlightenment.

17. What "ideological principle" is the author referring to in the middle of the second paragraph when talking about the "Friar's Tale"?
    a. The principle that the act of ravaging another's possessions is the same as ravaging one's soul.
    b. The principle that thieves who idolize physical wealth will be punished in an earthly sense as well as eternally.
    c. The principle that fraternization with a demon will result in one losing everything, including his or her life.
    d. The principle that a desire for material goods leads to moral malfeasance punishable by a higher being.

18. Which of the following words, if substituted for the word *avarice* in paragraph two, would LEAST change the meaning of the sentence?
    a. Perniciousness
    b. Pithiness
    c. Parsimoniousness
    d. Precariousness

19. Based on the passage, what view does Boethianism take on desire?
    a. Desire does not exist in the context of Boethianism
    b. Desire is a virtue and should be welcomed
    c. Having desire is evidence of demonic possession
    d. Desire for pleasure can lead toward sin

Questions 20-27 are based on the following passages:

Passage I

Lethal force, or deadly force, is defined as the physical means to cause death or serious harm to another individual. The law holds that lethal force is only accepted when you or another person are in immediate and unavoidable danger of death or severe bodily harm. For example, a person could be beating a weaker person in such a way that they are suffering severe enough trauma that could result in death or serious harm. This would be an instance where lethal force would be acceptable and possibly the only way to save that person from irrevocable damage.

Another example of when to use lethal force would be when someone enters your home with a deadly weapon. The intruder's presence and possession of the weapon indicate mal-intent and the ability to inflict death or severe injury to you and your loved ones. Again, lethal force can be used in this situation. Lethal force can also be applied to prevent the harm of another individual. If a woman is being brutally assaulted and is unable to fend off an attacker, lethal force can be used to defend her as a last-ditch effort. If she is in immediate jeopardy of rape, harm, and/or death, lethal force could be the only response that could effectively deter the assailant.

The key to understanding the concept of lethal force is the term *last resort*. Deadly force cannot be taken back; it should be used only to prevent severe harm or death. The law does distinguish whether the means of one's self-defense is fully warranted, or if the individual goes out of control in the process. If you continually attack the assailant after they are rendered incapacitated, this would be causing unnecessary harm, and the law can bring charges against you. Likewise, if you kill an attacker unnecessarily after defending yourself, you can be charged with murder. This would move lethal force beyond necessary defense, making it no longer a last resort but rather a use of excessive force.

Passage II

Assault is the unlawful attempt of one person to apply apprehension on another individual by an imminent threat or by initiating offensive contact. Assaults can vary, encompassing physical strikes, threatening body language, and even provocative language. In the case of the latter, even if a hand has not been laid, it is still considered an assault because of its threatening nature.

Let's look at an example: A homeowner is angered because his neighbor blows fallen leaves into his freshly mowed lawn. Irate, the homeowner gestures a fist to his fellow neighbor and threatens to bash his head in for littering on his lawn. The homeowner's physical motions and verbal threat heralds a physical threat against the other neighbor. These factors classify the homeowner's reaction as an assault. If the angry neighbor hits the threatening homeowner in retaliation, that would constitute an assault as well because he physically hit the homeowner.

Assault also centers on the involvement of weapons in a conflict. If someone fires a gun at another person, this could be interpreted as an assault unless the shooter acted in self-defense. If an individual drew a gun or a knife on someone with the intent to harm them, that would be considered assault. However, it's also considered an assault if someone simply aimed a weapon, loaded or not, at another person in a threatening manner.

20. What is the purpose of the second passage?
   a. To inform the reader about what assault is and how it is committed
   b. To inform the reader about how assault is a minor example of lethal force
   c. To disprove the previous passage concerning lethal force
   d. The author is recounting an incident in which they were assaulted

21. Which of the following situations, according to the passages, would not constitute an illegal use of lethal force?
   a. A disgruntled cash register yells obscenities at a customer.
   b. A thief is seen running away with stolen cash.
   c. A man is attacked in an alley by another man with a knife.
   d. A woman punches another woman in a bar.

22. Given the information in the passages, which of the following must be true about assault?
   a. Assault charges are more severe than unnecessary use of force charges.
   b. There are various forms of assault.
   c. Smaller, weaker people cannot commit assaults.
   d. Assault is justified only as a last resort.

23. Which of the following, if true, would most seriously undermine the explanation proposed by the author in Passage I in the third paragraph?
   a. An instance of lethal force in self-defense is not absolutely absolved from blame. The law considers the necessary use of force at the time it is committed.
   b. An individual who uses lethal force under necessary defense is in direct compliance of the law under most circumstances.
   c. Lethal force in self-defense should be forgiven in all cases for the peace of mind of the primary victim.
   d. The use of lethal force is not evaluated on the intent of the user, but rather the severity of the primary attack that warranted self-defense.

24. Based on the passages, what can be inferred about the relationship between assault and lethal force?
   a. An act of lethal force always leads to a type of assault.
   b. An assault will result in someone using lethal force.
   c. An assault with deadly intent can lead to an individual using lethal force to preserve their well-being.
   d. If someone uses self-defense in a conflict, it is called deadly force; if actions or threats are intended, it is called assault.

25. Which of the following best describes the way the passages are structured?
   a. Both passages open by defining a legal concept and then continue to describe situations that further explain the concept.
   b. Both passages begin with situations, introduce accepted definitions, and then cite legal ramifications.
   c. Passage I presents a long definition while the Passage II begins by showing an example of assault.
   d. Both cite specific legal doctrines, then proceed to explain the rulings.

26. What can be inferred about the role of intent in lethal force and assault?
   a. Intent is irrelevant. The law does not take intent into account.
   b. Intent is vital for determining the lawfulness of using lethal force.
   c. Intent is very important for determining both lethal force and assault; intent is examined in both parties and helps determine the severity of the issue.
   d. The intent of the assailant is the main focus for determining legal ramifications; it is used to determine if the defender was justified in using force to respond.

27. The author uses the example in the second paragraph of Passage II in order to do what?
   a. To demonstrate two different types of assault by showing how each specifically relates to the other
   b. To demonstrate a single example of two different types of assault, then adding in the third type of assault in the example's conclusion
   c. To prove that the definition of lethal force is altered when the victim in question is a homeowner and his property is threatened
   d. To suggest that verbal assault can be an exaggerated crime by the law and does not necessarily lead to physical violence

Questions 28-33 are based upon the following passage:

> This excerpt is adapted from "What to the Slave is the Fourth of July?" Rochester, New York July 5, 1852.
>
> Fellow citizens—Pardon me, and allow me to ask, why am I called upon to speak here today? What have I, or those I represent, to do with your national independence? Are the great principles of political freedom and of natural justice embodied in that Declaration of Independence, Independence extended to us? And am I therefore called upon to bring our humble offering to the national altar, and to confess the benefits, and express devout gratitude for the blessings, resulting from your independence to us?
>
> Would to God, both for your sakes and ours, ours that an affirmative answer could be truthfully returned to these questions! Then would my task be light, and my burden easy and delightful. For who is there so cold that a nation's sympathy could not warm him? Who so obdurate and dead to the claims of gratitude, gratitude that that would not thankfully acknowledge such priceless benefits? Who so stolid and selfish, that would not give his voice to swell the hallelujahs of a nation's jubilee, when the chains of servitude had been torn from his limbs? I am not that man. In a case like that, the dumb my eloquently speak, and the lame man leap as an hart.
>
> But, such is not the state of the case. I say it with a sad sense of the disparity between us. I am not included within the pale of this glorious and anniversary. Oh pity! Your high independence only reveals the immeasurable distance between us. The blessings in

which you this day rejoice, I do not enjoy in common. The rich inheritance of justice, liberty, prosperity, and independence, bequeathed by your fathers, is shared by *you*, not by *me*. This Fourth of July is *yours,* not *mine*. You may rejoice, *I* must mourn. To drag a man in fetters into the grand illuminated temple of liberty, and call upon him to join you in joyous anthems, were inhuman mockery and sacrilegious irony. Do you mean, citizens, to mock me, by asking me to speak today? If so there is a parallel to your conduct. And let me warn you that it is dangerous to copy the example of a nation whose crimes, towering up to heaven, were thrown down by the breath of the Almighty, burying that nation and irrecoverable ruin! I can today take up the plaintive lament of a peeled and woe-smitten people.

By the rivers of Babylon, there we sat down. Yea! We wept when we remembered Zion. We hanged our harps upon the willows in the midst thereof. For there, they that carried us away captive, required of us a song; and they who wasted us required of us mirth, saying, "Sing us one of the songs of Zion." How can we sing the Lord's song in a strange land? If I forget thee, O Jerusalem, let my right hand forget her cunning. If I do not remember thee, let my tongue cleave to the roof of my mouth.

28. What is the tone of the first paragraph of this passage?
   a. Exasperated
   b. Inclusive
   c. Contemplative
   d. Nonchalant

29. Which word CANNOT be used synonymously with the term *obdurate* as it is conveyed in the text below?

   Who so obdurate and dead to the claims of gratitude, that would not thankfully acknowledge such priceless benefits?

   a. Steadfast
   b. Stubborn
   c. Contented
   d. Unwavering

30. What is the central purpose of this text?
   a. To demonstrate the author's extensive knowledge of the Bible
   b. To address the feelings of exclusion expressed by African Americans after the establishment of the Fourth of July holiday
   c. To convince wealthy landowners to adopt new holiday rituals
   d. To explain why minorities often relished the notion of segregation in government institutions

31. Which statement serves as evidence for the question above?
   a. By the rivers of Babylon...down.
   b. Fellow citizens...today.
   c. I can...woe-smitten people.
   d. The rich inheritance of justice...*not by me*.

32. The statement below features an example of which of the following literary devices?
    Oh pity! Your high independence only reveals the immeasurable distance between us.

   a. Assonance
   b. Parallelism
   c. Amplification
   d. Hyperbole

33. The speaker's use of biblical references, such as "rivers of Babylon" and the "songs of Zion," helps the reader to do all EXCEPT which of the following?
   a. Identify with the speaker using common text
   b. Convince the audience that injustices have been committed by referencing another group of people who have been previously affected by slavery
   c. Display the equivocation of the speaker and those that he represents
   d. Appeal to the listener's sense of humanity

Questions 34-39 are based upon the following passage:

> This excerpt is adaptation from Abraham Lincoln's Address Delivered at the Dedication of the Cemetery at Gettysburg, November 19, 1863.
>
> Four score and seven years ago our fathers brought forth on this continent, a new nation, conceived in liberty, and dedicated to the proposition that all men are created equal.
>
> Now we are engaged in a great civil war, testing whether that nation, or any nation so conceived and so dedicated, can long endure. We are met on a great battlefield of that war. We have come to dedicate a portion of that field, as a final resting place for those who here gave their lives that this nation might live. It is altogether fitting and proper that we should do this.
>
> But, in a larger sense, we cannot dedicate—we cannot consecrate that we cannot hallow—this ground. The brave men, living and dead, who struggled here, have consecrated it, far above our poor power to add or detract. The world will little note, nor long remember what we say here, but it can never forget what they did here. It is for us the living, rather, to be dedicated here to the unfinished work which they who fought here have thus far so nobly advanced. It is rather for us to be here and dedicated to the great task remaining before us—that from these honored dead we take increased devotion to that cause for which they gave the last full measure of devotion—that we here highly resolve that these dead shall not have died in vain—that these this nation, under God, shall have a new birth of freedom—and that government of people, by the people, for the people, shall not perish from the earth.

34. The best description for the phrase *four score and seven years ago* is which of the following?
   a. A unit of measurement
   b. A period of time
   c. A literary movement
   d. A statement of political reform

35. What is the setting of this text?
    a. A battleship off of the coast of France
    b. A desert plain on the Sahara Desert
    c. A battlefield in North America
    d. The residence of Abraham Lincoln

36. Which war is Abraham Lincoln referring to in the following passage?
    > Now we are engaged in a great civil war, testing whether that nation, or any nation so conceived and so dedicated, can long endure.

    a. World War I
    b. The War of the Spanish Succession
    c. World War II
    d. The American Civil War

37. What message is the author trying to convey through this address?
    a. The audience should consider the death of the people that fought in the war as an example and perpetuate the ideals of freedom that the soldiers died fighting for.
    b. The audience should honor the dead by establishing an annual memorial service.
    c. The audience should form a militia that would overturn the current political structure.
    d. The audience should forget the lives that were lost and discredit the soldiers.

38. Which rhetorical device is being used in the following passage?
    > ...we here highly resolve that these dead shall not have died in vain—that these this nation, under God, shall have a new birth of freedom—and that government of people, by the people, for the people, shall not perish from the earth.

    a. Antimetatabolee
    b. Antiphrasis
    c. Anaphora
    d. Epiphora

39. What is the effect of Lincoln's statement in the following passage?
    > But, in a larger sense, we cannot dedicate—we cannot consecrate that we cannot hallow—this ground. The brave men, living and dead, who struggled here, have consecrated it, far above our poor power to add or detract.

    a. His comparison emphasizes the great sacrifice of the soldiers who fought in the war.
    b. His comparison serves as a remainder of the inadequacies of his audience.
    c. His comparison serves as a catalyst for guilt and shame among audience members.
    d. His comparison attempts to illuminate the great differences between soldiers and civilians.

Questions 40-45 are based upon the following passage:

This excerpt is adaptation from Charles Dickens' speech in Birmingham in England on December 30, 1853 on behalf of the Birmingham and Midland Institute.

My Good Friends,—When I first imparted to the committee of the projected Institute my particular wish that on one of the evenings of my readings here the main body of my audience should be composed of working men and their families, I was animated by two desires; first, by the wish to have the great pleasure of meeting you face to face at this Christmas time, and accompany you myself through one of my little Christmas books; and second, by the wish to have an opportunity of stating publicly in your presence, and in the presence of the committee, my earnest hope that the Institute will, from the beginning, recognise one great principle—strong in reason and justice—which I believe to be essential to the very life of such an Institution. It is, that the working man shall, from the first unto the last, have a share in the management of an Institution which is designed for his benefit, and which calls itself by his name.

I have no fear here of being misunderstood—of being supposed to mean too much in this. If there ever was a time when any one class could of itself do much for its own good, and for the welfare of society—which I greatly doubt—that time is unquestionably past. It is in the fusion of different classes, without confusion; in the bringing together of employers and employed; in the creating of a better common understanding among those whose interests are identical, who depend upon each other, who are vitally essential to each other, and who never can be in unnatural antagonism without deplorable results, that one of the chief principles of a Mechanics' Institution should consist. In this world, a great deal of the bitterness among us arises from an imperfect understanding of one another. Erect in Birmingham a great Educational Institution, properly educational; educational of the feelings as well as of the reason; to which all orders of Birmingham men contribute; in which all orders of Birmingham men meet; wherein all orders of Birmingham men are faithfully represented—and you will erect a Temple of Concord here which will be a model edifice to the whole of England.

Contemplating as I do the existence of the Artisans' Committee, which not long ago considered the establishment of the Institute so sensibly, and supported it so heartily, I earnestly entreat the gentlemen—earnest I know in the good work, and who are now among us—by all means to avoid the great shortcoming of similar institutions; and in asking the working man for his confidence, to set him the great example and give him theirs in return. You will judge for yourselves if I promise too much for the working man, when I say that he will stand by such an enterprise with the utmost of his patience, his perseverance, sense, and support; that I am sure he will need no charitable aid or condescending patronage; but will readily and cheerfully pay for the advantages which it confers; that he will prepare himself in individual cases where he feels that the adverse circumstances around him have rendered it necessary; in a word, that he will feel his responsibility like an honest man, and will most honestly and manfully discharge it. I now proceed to the pleasant task to which I assure you I have looked forward for a long time.

40. Which word is most closely synonymous with the word *patronage* as it appears in the following statement?
    ...that I am sure he will need no charitable aid or condescending patronage

    a. Auspices
    b. Aberration
    c. Acerbic
    d. Adulation

41. Which term is most closely aligned with the definition of the term *working man* as it is defined in the following passage?

> You will judge for yourselves if I promise too much for the working man, when I say that he will stand by such an enterprise with the utmost of his patience, his perseverance, sense, and support...

    a. Plebian
    b. Viscount
    c. Entrepreneur
    d. Bourgeois

42. Which of the following statements most closely correlates with the definition of the term *working man* as it is defined in Question 41?
    a. A working man is not someone who works for institutions or corporations, but someone who is well-versed in the workings of the soul.
    b. A working man is someone who is probably not involved in social activities because the physical demand for work is too high.
    c. A working man is someone who works for wages among the middle class.
    d. The working man has historically taken to the field, to the factory, and now to the screen.

43. Based upon the contextual evidence provided in the passage above, what is the meaning of the term *enterprise* in the third paragraph?
    a. Company
    b. Courage
    c. Game
    d. Cause

44. The speaker addresses his audience as *My Good Friends.* What kind of credibility does this salutation give to the speaker?
    a. The speaker is an employer addressing his employees, so the salutation is a way for the boss to bridge the gap between himself and his employees.
    b. The speaker's salutation is one from an entertainer to his audience, and uses the friendly language to connect to his audience before a serious speech.
    c. The salutation is used ironically to give a somber tone to the serious speech that follows.
    d. The speech is one from a politician to the public, so the salutation is used to grab the audience's attention.

45. According to the passage, what is the speaker's second desire for his time in front of the audience?
    a. To read a Christmas story
    b. For the working man to have a say in his institution, which is designed for his benefit.
    c. To have an opportunity to stand in their presence
    d. For the life of the institution to be essential to the audience as a whole

Questions 46-51 are based upon the following passage:

> "MANKIND being originally equals in the order of creation, the equality could only be destroyed by some subsequent circumstance; the distinctions of rich, and poor, may in a great measure be accounted for, and that without having recourse to the harsh ill sounding names of oppression and avarice. Oppression is often the consequence, but

69

seldom or never the means of riches; and though avarice will preserve a man from being necessitously poor, it generally makes him too timorous to be wealthy.

But there is another and greater distinction for which no truly natural or religious reason can be assigned, and that is, the distinction of men into KINGS and SUBJECTS. Male and female are the distinctions of nature, good and bad the distinctions of heaven; but how a race of men came into the world so exalted above the rest, and distinguished like some new species, is worth enquiring into, and whether they are the means of happiness or of misery to mankind.

In the early ages of the world, according to the scripture chronology, there were no kings; the consequence of which was there were no wars; it is the pride of kings which throw mankind into confusion Holland without a king hath enjoyed more peace for this last century than any of the monarchical governments in Europe. Antiquity favors the same remark; for the quiet and rural lives of the first patriarchs hath a happy something in them, which vanishes away when we come to the history of Jewish royalty.

Government by kings was first introduced into the world by the Heathens, from whom the children of Israel copied the custom. It was the most prosperous invention the Devil ever set on foot for the promotion of idolatry. The Heathens paid divine honors to their deceased kings, and the Christian world hath improved on the plan by doing the same to their living ones. How impious is the title of sacred majesty applied to a worm, who in the midst of his splendor is crumbling into dust!

As the exalting one man so greatly above the rest cannot be justified on the equal rights of nature, so neither can it be defended on the authority of scripture; for the will of the Almighty, as declared by Gideon and the prophet Samuel, expressly disapproves of government by kings. All anti-monarchical parts of scripture have been very smoothly glossed over in monarchical governments, but they undoubtedly merit the attention of countries, which have their governments yet to form. "Render unto Caesar the things which are Caesar's" is the scripture doctrine of courts, yet it is no support of monarchical government, for the Jews at that time were without a king, and in a state of vassalage to the Romans.

Near three thousand years passed away from the Mosaic account of the creation, till the Jews under a national delusion requested a king. Till then their form of government (except in extraordinary cases, where the Almighty interposed) was a kind of republic administered by a judge and the elders of the tribes. Kings they had none, and it was held sinful to acknowledge any being under that title but the Lord of Hosts. And when a man seriously reflects on the idolatrous homage which is paid to the persons of Kings, he need not wonder, that the Almighty ever jealous of his honor, should disapprove of a form of government which so impiously invades the prerogative of heaven.

Excerpt From: Thomas Paine. "Common Sense."

46. According to passage, what role does avarice, or greed, play in poverty?
    a. It can make a man very wealthy
    b. It is the consequence of wealth
    c. Avarice can prevent a man from being poor, but too fearful to be very wealthy
    d. Avarice is what drives a person to be very wealthy

47. Of these distinctions, which does the author believe to be beyond natural or religious reason?
    a. Good and bad
    b. Male and female
    c. Human and animal
    d. King and subjects

48. According to the passage, what are the Heathens responsible for?
    a. Government by kings
    b. Quiet and rural lives of patriarchs
    c. Paying divine honors to their living kings
    d. Equal rights of nature

49. Which of the following best states Paine's rationale for the denouncement of monarchy?
    a. It is against the laws of nature
    b. It is against the equal rights of nature and is denounced in scripture
    c. Despite scripture, a monarchal government is unlawful
    d. Neither the law nor scripture denounce monarchy

50. Based on the passage, what is the best definition of the word *idolatrous*?
    a. Worshipping heroes
    b. Being deceitful
    c. Sinfulness
    d. Engaging in illegal activities

51. What is the essential meaning of lines 41-44?
    And when a man seriously reflects on the idolatrous homage which is paid to the persons of Kings, he need not wonder, that the Almighty ever jealous of his honor, should disapprove of a form of government which so impiously invades the prerogative of heaven.

    a. God would disapprove of the irreverence of a monarchical government.
    b. With careful reflection, men should realize that heaven is not promised.
    c. God will punish those that follow a monarchical government.
    d. Belief in a monarchical government cannot coexist with belief in God.

Questions 52-57 are based upon the following passage:

This excerpt is an adaptation of Jonathan Swift's *Gulliver's Travels into Several Remote Nations of the World.*

My gentleness and good behaviour had gained so far on the emperor and his court, and indeed upon the army and people in general, that I began to conceive hopes of getting my liberty in a short time. I took all possible methods to cultivate this favourable disposition. The natives came, by degrees, to be less apprehensive of any danger from me. I would sometimes lie down, and let five or six of them dance on my hand; and at last the boys and girls would venture to come and play at hide-and-seek in my hair. I had now made a good progress in understanding and speaking the language. The emperor had a mind one day to entertain me with several of the country shows, wherein they exceed all nations I have known, both for dexterity and magnificence. I was diverted with none so much as that of the rope-dancers, performed upon a slender white thread, extended about two feet, and twelve inches from the ground. Upon which I shall desire liberty, with the reader's patience, to enlarge a little.

This diversion is only practised by those persons who are candidates for great employments, and high favour at court. They are trained in this art from their youth, and are not always of noble birth, or liberal education. When a great office is vacant, either by death or disgrace (which often happens,) five or six of those candidates petition the emperor to entertain his majesty and the court with a dance on the rope; and whoever jumps the highest, without falling, succeeds in the office. Very often the chief ministers themselves are commanded to show their skill, and to convince the emperor that they have not lost their faculty. Flimnap, the treasurer, is allowed to cut a caper on the straight rope, at least an inch higher than any other lord in the whole empire. I have seen him do the summerset several times together, upon a trencher fixed on a rope which is no thicker than a common packthread in England. My friend Reldresal, principal secretary for private affairs, is, in my opinion, if I am not partial, the second after the treasurer; the rest of the great officers are much upon a par.

52. Which of the following statements best summarize the central purpose of this text?
    a. Gulliver details his fondness for the archaic yet interesting practices of his captors.
    b. Gulliver conjectures about the intentions of the aristocratic sector of society.
    c. Gulliver becomes acquainted with the people and practices of his new surroundings.
    d. Gulliver's differences cause him to become penitent around new acquaintances.

53. What is the word *principal* referring to in the following text?
    My friend Reldresal, principal secretary for private affairs, is, in my opinion, if I am not partial, the second after the treasurer; the rest of the great officers are much upon a par.

    a. Primary or chief
    b. An acolyte
    c. An individual who provides nurturing
    d. One in a subordinate position

54. What can the reader infer from this passage?
    I would sometimes lie down, and let five or six of them dance on my hand; and at last the boys and girls would venture to come and play at hide-and-seek in my hair.

    a. The children tortured Gulliver.
    b. Gulliver traveled because he wanted to meet new people.
    c. Gulliver is considerably larger than the children who are playing around him.
    d. Gulliver has a genuine love and enthusiasm for people of all sizes.

55. What is the significance of the word *mind* in the following passage?
    The emperor had a mind one day to entertain me with several of the country shows, wherein they exceed all nations I have known, both for dexterity and magnificence.

    a. The ability to think
    b. A collective vote
    c. A definitive decision
    d. A mythological question

56. Which of the following assertions does not support the fact that games are a commonplace event in this culture?
   a. My gentlest and good behavior . . . short time.
   b. They are trained in this art from their youth . . . liberal education.
   c. Very often the chief ministers themselves are commanded to show their skill . . . not lost their faculty.
   d. Flimnap, the treasurer, is allowed to cut a caper on the straight rope . . . higher than any other lord in the whole empire.

57. How does Gulliver's description of Flimnap's, the treasurer's, ability to *cut a caper on the straight rope*, and Reldresal, principal secretary for private affairs, being the *second to the treasurer,* serve as evidence of the community's emphasis in regards to the correlation between physical strength and leadership abilities?
   a. Only children used Gulliver's hands as a playground.
   b. The two men who exhibited superior abilities held prominent positions in the community.
   c. Only common townspeople, not leaders, walk the straight rope.
   d. No one could jump higher than Gulliver.

Questions 58-63 are based upon the following passage:

This excerpt is adaptation of Robert Louis Stevenson's *The Strange Case of Dr. Jekyll and Mr. Hyde.*

"Did you ever come across a protégé of his—one Hyde?" He asked.

"Hyde?" repeated Lanyon. "No. Never heard of him. Since my time."

That was the amount of information that the lawyer carried back with him to the great, dark bed on which he tossed to and fro until the small hours of the morning began to grow large. It was a night of little ease to his toiling mind, toiling in mere darkness and besieged by questions.

Six o'clock struck on the bells of the church that was so conveniently near to Mr. Utterson's dwelling, and still he was digging at the problem. Hitherto it had touched him on the intellectual side alone; but; but now his imagination also was engaged, or rather enslaved; and as he lay and tossed in the gross darkness of the night in the curtained room, Mr. Enfield's tale went by before his mind in a scroll of lighted pictures. He would be aware of the great field of lamps in a nocturnal city; then of the figure of a man walking swiftly; then of a child running from the doctor's; and then these met, and that human Juggernaut trod the child down and passed on regardless of her screams. Or else he would see a room in a rich house, where his friend lay asleep, dreaming and smiling at his dreams; and then the door of that room would be opened, the curtains of the bed plucked apart, the sleeper recalled, and, lo! There would stand by his side a figure to whom power was given, and even at that dead hour he must rise and do its bidding. The figure in these two phrases haunted the lawyer all night; and if at anytime he dozed over, it was but to see it glide more stealthily through sleeping houses, or move the more swiftly, and still the more smoothly, even to dizziness, through wider labyrinths of lamplighted city, and at every street corner crush a child and leave her screaming. And still the figure had no face by which he might know it; even in his dreams it had no face, or one that baffled him and melted before his eyes; and thus there it was that there sprung up and grew apace in the lawyer's mind a singularly strong, almost an inordinate, curiosity to behold the features of the real Mr. Hyde. If he could but once set eyes on him, he thought the mystery would lighten and perhaps roll altogether away, as was the habit of mysterious things when well examined. He might see a reason for his friend's strange preference or bondage, and even for the startling clauses of the will. And at least it would be a face worth seeing: the face of a man who was without bowels of mercy: a face which had but to show itself to raise up, in the mind of the unimpressionable Enfield, a spirit of enduring hatred.

From that time forward, Mr. Utterson began to haunt the door in the by street of shops. In the morning before office hours, at noon when business was plenty of time scares, at night under the face of the full city moon, by all lights and at all hours of solitude or concourse, the lawyer was to be found on his chosen post.

"If he be Mr. Hyde," he had thought, "I should be Mr. Seek."

58. What is the purpose of the use of repetition in the following passage?
    It was a night of little ease to his toiling mind, toiling in mere darkness and besieged by questions.

    a. It serves as a demonstration of the mental state of Mr. Lanyon.
    b. It is reminiscent of the church bells that are mentioned in the story.
    c. It mimics Mr. Utterson's ambivalence.
    d. It emphasizes Mr. Utterson's anguish in failing to identify Hyde's whereabouts.

59. What is the setting of the story in this passage?
    a. In the city
    b. On the countryside
    c. In a jail
    d. In a mental health facility

60. What can one infer about the meaning of the word "Juggernaut" from the author's use of it in the passage?
    a. It is an apparition that appears at daybreak.
    b. It scares children.
    c. It is associated with space travel.
    d. Mr. Utterson finds it soothing.

61. What is the definition of the word *haunt* in the following passage?
    From that time forward, Mr. Utterson began to haunt the door in the by street of shops. In the morning before office hours, at noon when business was plenty of time scares, at night under the face of the full city moon, by all lights and at all hours of solitude or concourse, the lawyer was to be found on his chosen post.

    a. To levitate
    b. To constantly visit
    c. To terrorize
    d. To daunt

62. The phrase *labyrinths of lamplighted city* contains an example of what?
    a. Hyperbole
    b. Simile
    c. Metaphor
    d. Alliteration

63. What can one reasonably conclude from the final comment of this passage?
    "If he be Mr. Hyde," he had thought, "I should be Mr. Seek."

    a. The speaker is considering a name change.
    b. The speaker is experiencing an identity crisis.
    c. The speaker has mistakenly been looking for the wrong person.
    d. The speaker intends to continue to look for Hyde.

Questions 64-69 are based upon the following passage:

This excerpt is adaptation from *Our Vanishing Wildlife,* by William T. Hornaday

> Three years ago, I think there were not many bird-lovers in the United States, who believed it possible to prevent the total extinction of both egrets from our fauna. All the known rookeries accessible to plume-hunters had been totally destroyed. Two years ago, the secret discovery of several small, hidden colonies prompted William Dutcher, President of the National Association of Audubon Societies, and Mr. T. Gilbert Pearson, Secretary, to attempt the protection of those colonies. With a fund contributed for the purpose, wardens were hired and duly commissioned. As previously stated, one of those wardens was shot dead in cold blood by a plume hunter. The task of guarding swamp rookeries from the attacks of money-hungry desperadoes to whom the accursed plumes were worth their weight in gold, is a very chancy proceeding. There is now one warden in Florida who says that "before they get my rookery they will first have to get me."

> Thus far the protective work of the Audubon Association has been successful. Now there are twenty colonies, which contain all told, about 5,000 egrets and about 120,000 herons and ibises which are guarded by the Audubon wardens. One of the most important is on Bird Island, a mile out in Orange Lake, central Florida, and it is ably defended by Oscar E. Baynard. To-day, the plume hunters who do not dare to raid the guarded rookeries are trying to study out the lines of flight of the birds, to and from their feeding-grounds, and shoot them in transit. Their motto is—"Anything to beat the law, and get the plumes." It is there that the state of Florida should take part in the war.

> The success of this campaign is attested by the fact that last year a number of egrets were seen in eastern Massachusetts—for the first time in many years. And so to-day the question is, can the wardens continue to hold the plume-hunters at bay?

64. The author's use of first person pronoun in the following text does NOT have which of the following effects?

> Three years ago, I think there were not many bird-lovers in the United States, who believed it possible to prevent the total extinction of both egrets from our fauna.

a. The phrase *I think* acts as a sort of hedging, where the author's tone is less direct and/or absolute.
b. It allows the reader to more easily connect with the author.
c. It encourages the reader to empathize with the egrets.
d. It distances the reader from the text by overemphasizing the story.

65. What purpose does the quote serve at the end of the first paragraph?
a. The quote shows proof of a hunter threatening one of the wardens.
b. The quote lightens the mood by illustrating the colloquial language of the region.
c. The quote provides an example of a warden protecting one of the colonies.
d. The quote provides much needed comic relief in the form of a joke.

66. What is the meaning of the word *rookeries* in the following text?

> To-day, the plume hunters who do not dare to raid the guarded rookeries are trying to study out the lines of flight of the birds, to and from their feeding-grounds, and shoot them in transit.

a. Houses in a slum area
b. A place where hunters gather to trade tools
c. A place where wardens go to trade stories
d. A colony of breeding birds

67. What is on Bird Island?
a. Hunters selling plumes
b. An important bird colony
c. Bird Island Battle between the hunters and the wardens
d. An important egret with unique plumes

68. What is the main purpose of the passage?
a. To persuade the audience to act in preservation of the bird colonies
b. To show the effect hunting egrets has had on the environment
c. To argue that the preservation of bird colonies has had a negative impact on the environment.
d. To demonstrate the success of the protective work of the Audubon Association

69. Why are hunters trying to study the lines of flight of the birds?
a. To study ornithology, one must know the lines of flight that birds take.
b. To help wardens preserve the lives of the birds
c. To have a better opportunity to hunt the birds
d. To builds their homes under the lines of flight because they believe it brings good luck

Questions 70-75 are based upon the following passage:

This excerpt is adaptation from *The Life-Story of Insects,* by Geo H. Carpenter.

> Insects as a whole are preeminently creatures of the land and the air. This is shown not only by the possession of wings by a vast majority of the class, but by the mode of breathing to which reference has already been made, a system of branching air-tubes

76

carrying atmospheric air with its combustion-supporting oxygen to all the insect's tissues. The air gains access to these tubes through a number of paired air-holes or spiracles, arranged segmentally in series.

It is of great interest to find that, nevertheless, a number of insects spend much of their time under water. This is true of not a few in the perfect winged state, as for example aquatic beetles and water-bugs ('boatmen' and 'scorpions') which have some way of protecting their spiracles when submerged, and, possessing usually the power of flight, can pass on occasion from pond or stream to upper air. But it is advisable in connection with our present subject to dwell especially on some insects that remain continually under water till they are ready to undergo their final moult and attain the winged state, which they pass entirely in the air. The preparatory instars of such insects are aquatic; the adult instar is aerial. All may-flies, dragon-flies, and caddis-flies, many beetles and two-winged flies, and a few moths thus divide their life-story between the water and the air. For the present we confine attention to the Stone-flies, the May-flies, and the Dragon-flies, three well-known orders of insects respectively called by systematists the Plecoptera, the Ephemeroptera and the Odonata.

In the case of many insects that have aquatic larvae, the latter are provided with some arrangement for enabling them to reach atmospheric air through the surface-film of the water. But the larva of a stone-fly, a dragon-fly, or a may-fly is adapted more completely than these for aquatic life; it can, by means of gills of some kind, breathe the air dissolved in water.

70. Which statement best details the central idea in this passage?
    a. It introduces certain insects that transition from water to air.
    b. It delves into entomology, especially where gills are concerned.
    c. It defines what constitutes as insects' breathing.
    d. It invites readers to have a hand in the preservation of insects.

71. Which definition most closely relates to the usage of the word *moult* in the passage?
    a. An adventure of sorts, especially underwater
    b. Mating act between two insects
    c. The act of shedding part or all of the outer shell
    d. Death of an organism that ends in a revival of life

72. What is the purpose of the first paragraph in relation to the second paragraph?
    a. The first paragraph serves as a cause and the second paragraph serves as an effect.
    b. The first paragraph serves as a contrast to the second.
    c. The first paragraph is a description for the argument in the second paragraph.
    d. The first and second paragraphs are merely presented in a sequence.

73. What does the following sentence most nearly mean?
    The preparatory instars of such insects are aquatic; the adult instar is aerial.

    a. The volume of water is necessary to prep the insect for transition rather than the volume of the air.
    b. The abdomen of the insect is designed like a star in the water as well as the air.
    c. The stage of preparation in between molting is acted out in the water, while the last stage is in the air.
    d. These insects breathe first in the water through gills, yet continue to use the same organs to breathe in the air.

74. Which of the statements reflect information that one could reasonably infer based on the author's tone?
    a. The author's tone is persuasive and attempts to call the audience to action.
    b. The author's tone is passionate due to excitement over the subject and personal narrative.
    c. The author's tone is informative and exhibits interest in the subject of the study.
    d. The author's tone is somber, depicting some anger at the state of insect larvae.

75. Which statement best describes stoneflies, mayflies, and dragonflies?
    a. They are creatures of the land and the air.
    b. They have a way of protecting their spiracles when submerged.
    c. Their larvae can breathe the air dissolved in water through gills of some kind.
    d. The preparatory instars of these insects are aerial.

Questions 76-80 are based upon the following passage:

This excerpt is adaptation from "The 'Hatchery' of the Sun-Fish"--- *Scientific American, #711*

> I have thought that an example of the intelligence (instinct?) of a class of fish which has come under my observation during my excursions into the Adirondack region of New York State might possibly be of interest to your readers, especially as I am not aware that any one except myself has noticed it, or, at least, has given it publicity.
>
> The female sun-fish (called, I believe, in England, the roach or bream) makes a "hatchery" for her eggs in this wise. Selecting a spot near the banks of the numerous lakes in which this region abounds, and where the water is about 4 inches deep, and still, she builds, with her tail and snout, a circular embankment 3 inches in height and 2 thick. The circle, which is as perfect a one as could be formed with mathematical instruments, is usually a foot and a half in diameter; and at one side of this circular wall an opening is left by the fish of just sufficient width to admit her body.
>
> The mother sun-fish, having now built or provided her "hatchery," deposits her spawn within the circular inclosure, and mounts guard at the entrance until the fry are hatched out and are sufficiently large to take charge of themselves. As the embankment, moreover, is built up to the surface of the water, no enemy can very easily obtain an entrance within the inclosure from the top; while there being only one entrance, the fish is able, with comparative ease, to keep out all intruders.

I have, as I say, noticed this beautiful instinct of the sun-fish for the perpetuity of her species more particularly in the lakes of this region; but doubtless the same habit is common to these fish in other waters.

76. What is the purpose of this passage?
    a. To show the effects of fish hatcheries on the Adirondack region
    b. To persuade the audience to study Ichthyology (fish science)
    c. To depict the sequence of mating among sun-fish
    d. To enlighten the audience on the habits of sun-fish and their hatcheries

77. What does the word *wise* in this passage most closely mean?
    a. Knowledge
    b. Manner
    c. Shrewd
    d. Ignorance

78. What is the definition of the word *fry* as it appears in the following passage?
    The mother sun-fish, having now built or provided her "hatchery," deposits her spawn within the circular inclosure, and mounts guard at the entrance until the fry are hatched out and are sufficiently large to take charge of themselves.

    a. Fish at the stage of development where they are capable of feeding themselves.
    b. Fish eggs that have been fertilized.
    c. A place where larvae is kept out of danger from other predators.
    d. A dish where fish is placed in oil and fried until golden brown.

79. How is the circle that keeps the larvae of the sun-fish made?
    a. It is formed with mathematical instruments.
    b. The sun-fish builds it with her tail and snout.
    c. It is provided to her as a "hatchery" by Mother Nature.
    d. The sun-fish builds it with her larvae.

80. The author included the third paragraph in the following passage to achieve which of the following effects?
    a. To complicate the subject matter
    b. To express a bias
    c. To insert a counterargument
    d. To conclude a sequence and add a final detail

Questions 81-86 are based on the following passage:

The following passage is an excerpt from *The Curious Case of Benjamin Button*, F.S. Fitzgerald, 1922

As long ago as 1860 it was the proper thing to be born at home. At present, so I am told, the high gods of medicine have decreed that the first cries of the young shall be uttered upon the anesthetic air of a hospital, preferably a fashionable one. So young Mr. and Mrs. Roger Button were fifty years ahead of style when they decided, one day in the summer of 1860, that their first baby should be born in a hospital. Whether this anachronism had any bearing upon the astonishing history I am about to set down will never be known.

I shall tell you what occurred, and let you judge for yourself.

The Roger Buttons held an enviable position, both social and financial, in ante-bellum Baltimore. They were related to the This Family and the That Family, which, as every Southerner knew, entitled them to membership in that enormous peerage which largely populated the Confederacy. This was their first experience with the charming old custom of having babies— Mr. Button was naturally nervous. He hoped it would be a boy so that he could be sent to Yale College in Connecticut, at which institution Mr. Button himself had been known for four years by the somewhat obvious nickname of "Cuff."

On the September morning <u>consecrated</u> to the enormous event he arose nervously at six o'clock dressed himself, adjusted an impeccable stock, and hurried forth through the streets of Baltimore to the hospital, to determine whether the darkness of the night had borne in new life upon its bosom.

When he was approximately a hundred yards from the Maryland Private Hospital for Ladies and Gentlemen he saw Doctor Keene, the family physician, descending the front steps, rubbing his hands together with a washing movement—as all doctors are required to do by the unwritten ethics of their profession.

Mr. Roger Button, the president of Roger Button & Co., Wholesale Hardware, began to run toward Doctor Keene with much less dignity than was expected from a Southern gentleman of that picturesque period. "Doctor Keene!" he called. "Oh, Doctor Keene!"

The doctor heard him, faced around, and stood waiting, a curious expression settling on his harsh, medicinal face as Mr. Button drew near.

"What happened?" demanded Mr. Button, as he came up in a gasping rush. "What was it? How is she? A boy? Who is it? What—"

"Talk sense!" said Doctor Keene sharply. He appeared somewhat irritated.

"Is the child born?" begged Mr. Button.

Doctor Keene frowned. "Why, yes, I suppose so—after a fashion." Again he threw a curious glance at Mr. Button.

81. What major event is about to happen in this story?
    a. Mr. Button is about to go to a funeral.
    b. Mr. Button's wife is about to have a baby.
    c. Mr. Button is getting ready to go to the doctor's office.
    d. Mr. Button is about to go shopping for new clothes.

82. What kind of tone does the above passage have?
    a. Nervous and Excited
    b. Sad and Angry
    c. Shameful and Confused
    d. Grateful and Joyous

83. What is the meaning of the word "consecrated" in paragraph 4?
    a. Numbed
    b. Chained
    c. Dedicated
    d. Moved

84. What does the author mean to do by adding the following statement?

    "rubbing his hands together with a washing movement—as all doctors are required to do by the unwritten ethics of their profession."

    a. Suggesting that Mr. Button is tired of the doctor.
    b. Trying to explain the detail of the doctor's profession.
    c. Hinting to readers that the doctor is an unethical man.
    d. Giving readers a visual picture of what the doctor is doing.

85. Which of the following best describes the development of this passage?
    a. It starts in the middle of a narrative in order to transition smoothly to a conclusion.
    b. It is a chronological narrative from beginning to end.
    c. The sequence of events is backwards—we go from future events to past events.
    d. To introduce the setting of the story and its characters.

86. Which of the following is an example of an imperative sentence?
    a. "Oh, Doctor Keene!"
    b. "Talk sense!"
    c. "Is the child born?"
    d. "Why, yes, I suppose so—"

Questions 87-92 are based on the following passage:

The following is an excerpt from "The Story of An Hour," Kate Chopin, 1894

> Knowing that Mrs. Mallard was afflicted with heart trouble, great care was taken to break to her as gently as possible the news of her husband's death.
>
> It was her sister Josephine who told her, in broken sentences; veiled hints that revealed in half concealing. Her husband's friend Richards was there, too, near her. It was he who had been in the newspaper office when intelligence of the railroad disaster was received, with Brently Mallard's name leading the list of "killed." He had only taken the time to assure himself of its truth by a second telegram, and had hastened to forestall any less careful, less tender friend in bearing the sad message.
>
> She did not hear the story as many women have heard the same, with a paralyzed inability to accept its significance. She wept at once, with sudden, wild abandonment, in her sister's arms. When the storm of grief had spent itself she went away to her room alone. She would have no one follow her.
>
> There stood, facing the open window, a comfortable, roomy armchair. Into this she sank, pressed down by a physical exhaustion that haunted her body and seemed to reach into her soul.

She could see in the open square before her house the tops of trees that were all aquiver with the new spring life. The delicious breath of rain was in the air. In the street below a peddler was crying his wares. The notes of a distant song which some one was singing reached her faintly, and countless sparrows were twittering in the eaves.

There were patches of blue sky showing here and there through the clouds that had met and piled one above the other in the west facing her window.

She sat with her head thrown back upon the cushion of the chair, quite motionless, except when a sob came up into her throat and shook her, as a child who has cried itself to sleep continues to sob in its dreams.

She was young, with a fair, calm face, whose lines bespoke repression and even a certain strength. But now here was a dull stare in her eyes, whose gaze was fixed away off yonder on one of those patches of blue sky. It was not a glance of reflection, but rather indicated a suspension of intelligent thought.

There was something coming to her and she was waiting for it, fearfully. What was it? She did not know; it was too subtle and elusive to name. But she felt it, creeping out of the sky, reaching toward her through the sounds, the scents, and color that filled the air.

Now her bosom rose and fell tumultuously. She was beginning to recognize this thing that was approaching to possess her, and she was striving to beat it back with her will—as powerless as her two white slender hands would have been. When she abandoned herself a little whispered word escaped her slightly parted lips. She said it over and over under her breath: "free, free, free!" The vacant stare and the look of terror that had followed it went from her eyes. They stayed keen and bright. Her pulses beat fast, and the coursing blood warmed and relaxed every inch of her body.

She did not stop to ask if it were or were not a monstrous joy that held her. A clear and exalted perception enabled her to dismiss the suggestion as trivial. She knew that she would weep again when she saw the kind, tender hands folded in death; the face that had never looked save with love upon her, fixed and gray and dead. But she saw beyond that bitter moment a long procession of years to come that would belong to her absolutely. And she opened and spread her arms out to them in welcome.

87. What point of view is the above passage told in?
    a. First person
    b. Second person
    c. Third person omniscient
    d. Third person limited

88. What kind of irony are we presented with in this story?
    a. The way Mrs. Mallard reacted to her husband's death.
    b. The way in which Mr. Mallard died.
    c. The way in which the news of her husband's death was presented to Mrs. Mallard.
    d. The way in which nature is compared with death in the story.

89. What is the meaning of the word "elusive" in paragraph 9?
    a. Horrible
    b. Indefinable
    c. Quiet
    d. Joyful

90. What is the best summary of the passage above?
    a. Mr. Mallard, a soldier during World War I, is killed by the enemy and leaves his wife widowed.
    b. Mrs. Mallard understands the value of friendship when her friends show up for her after her husband's death.
    c. Mrs. Mallard combats mental illness daily and will perhaps be sent to a mental institution soon.
    d. Mrs. Mallard, a newly widowed woman, finds unexpected relief in her husband's death.

91. What is the tone of this story?
    a. Confused
    b. Joyful
    c. Depressive
    d. All of the above

92. What is the meaning of the word "tumultuously" in paragraph 10?
    a. Orderly
    b. Unashamedly
    c. Violently
    d. Calmly

Questions 93-98 are based on the following passage:

This article discusses NASA technology.

When researchers and engineers undertake a large-scale scientific project, they may end up making discoveries and developing technologies that have far wider uses than originally intended. This is especially true in NASA, one of the most influential and innovative scientific organizations in America. NASA spinoff technology refers to innovations originally developed for NASA space projects that are now used in a wide range of different commercial fields. Many consumers are unaware that products they are buying are based on NASA research! Spinoff technology proves that it is worthwhile to invest in science research because it could enrich people's lives in unexpected ways.

The first spinoff technology worth mentioning is baby food. In space, where astronauts have limited access to fresh food and fewer options with their daily meals, malnutrition is a serious concern. Consequently, NASA researchers were looking for ways to enhance the nutritional value of astronauts' food. Scientists found that a certain type of algae could be added to food, improving the food's neurological benefits. When experts in the commercial food industry learned of this algae's potential to boost brain health, they were quick to begin their own research. The nutritional substance from algae then developed into a product called life's DHA, which can be found in over 90 percent of infant food sold in America.

Another intriguing example of a spinoff technology can be found in fashion. People who are always dropping their sunglasses may have invested in a pair of sunglasses with scratch resistant lenses—that is, it's impossible to scratch the glass, even if the glasses are dropped on an abrasive surface. This innovation is incredibly advantageous for people who are clumsy, but most shoppers don't know that this technology was originally developed by NASA. Scientists first created scratch resistant glass to help protect costly and crucial equipment from getting scratched in space, especially the helmet visors in space suits. However, sunglass companies later realized that this technology could be profitable for their products, and they licensed the technology from NASA.

93. What is the main purpose of this article?
    a. To advise consumers to do more research before making a purchase
    b. To persuade readers to support NASA research
    c. To tell a narrative about the history of space technology
    d. To define and describe instances of spinoff technology

94. What is the organizational structure of this article?
    a. A general definition followed by more specific examples
    b. A general opinion followed by supporting arguments
    c. An important moment in history followed by chronological details
    d. A popular misconception followed by counterevidence

95. Why did NASA scientists research algae?
    a. They already knew algae was healthy for babies.
    b. They were interested in how to grow food in space.
    c. They were looking for ways to add health benefits to food.
    d. They hoped to use it to protect expensive research equipment.

96. What does the word "neurological" mean in the second paragraph?
    a. Related to the body
    b. Related to the brain
    c. Related to vitamins
    d. Related to technology

97. Why does the author mention space suit helmets?
    a. To give an example of astronaut fashion
    b. To explain where sunglasses got their shape
    c. To explain how astronauts protect their eyes
    d. To give an example of valuable space equipment

98. Which statement would the author probably NOT agree with?
    a. Consumers don't always know the history of the products they are buying.
    b. Sometimes new innovations have unexpected applications.
    c. It is difficult to make money from scientific research.
    d. Space equipment is often very expensive.

Questions 99-103 are based on the following passage:

Christopher Columbus is often credited for discovering America. This is incorrect. First, it is impossible to "discover" something where people already live; however, Christopher Columbus did explore places in the New World that were previously untouched by Europe, so the term "explorer" would be more accurate. Another correction must be made, as well: Christopher Columbus was not the first European explorer to reach the present day Americas! Rather, it was

Leif Erikson who first came to the New World and contacted the natives, nearly five hundred years before Christopher Columbus.

Leif Erikson, the son of Erik the Red (a famous Viking outlaw and explorer in his own right), was born in either 970 or 980, depending on which historian you seek. His own family, though, did not raise Leif, which was a Viking tradition. Instead, one of Erik's prisoners taught Leif reading and writing, languages, sailing, and weaponry. At age 12, Leif was considered a man and returned to his family. He killed a man during a dispute shortly after his return, and the council banished the Erikson clan to Greenland.

In 999, Leif left Greenland and traveled to Norway where he would serve as a guard to King Olaf Tryggvason. It was there that he became a convert to Christianity. Leif later tried to return home with the intention of taking supplies and spreading Christianity to Greenland, however his ship was blown off course and he arrived in a strange new land: present day Newfoundland, Canada.

When he finally returned to his adopted homeland Greenland, Leif consulted with a merchant who had also seen the shores of this previously unknown land we now know as Canada. The son of the legendary Viking explorer then gathered a crew of 35 men and set sail. Leif became the first European to touch foot in the New World as he explored present-day Baffin Island and Labrador, Canada. His crew called the land Vinland since it was plentiful with grapes.

During their time in present-day Newfoundland, Leif's expedition made contact with the natives whom they referred to as Skraelings (which translates to "wretched ones" in Norse). There are several secondhand accounts of their meetings. Some contemporaries described trade between the peoples. Other accounts describe clashes where the Skraelings defeated the Viking explorers with long spears, while still others claim the Vikings dominated the natives. Regardless of the circumstances, it seems that the Vikings made contact of some kind. This happened around 1000, nearly five hundred years before Columbus famously sailed the ocean blue.

Eventually, in 1003, Leif set sail for home and arrived at Greenland with a ship full of timber.

In 1020, seventeen years later, the legendary Viking died. Many believe that Leif Erikson should receive more credit for his contributions in exploring the New World.

99. Which of the following best describes how the author generally presents the information?
   a. Chronological order
   b. Comparison-contrast
   c. Cause-effect
   d. Conclusion-premises

100. Which of the following is an opinion, rather than historical fact, expressed by the author?
   a. Leif Erikson was definitely the son of Erik the Red; however, historians debate the year of his birth.
   b. Leif Erikson's crew called the land Vinland since it was plentiful with grapes.
   c. Leif Erikson deserves more credit for his contributions in exploring the New World.
   d. Leif Erikson explored the Americas nearly five hundred years before Christopher Columbus.

101. Which of the following most accurately describes the author's main conclusion?
    a. Leif Erikson is a legendary Viking explorer.
    b. Leif Erikson deserves more credit for exploring America hundreds of years before Columbus.
    c. Spreading Christianity motivated Leif Erikson's expeditions more than any other factor.
    d. Leif Erikson contacted the natives nearly five hundred years before Columbus.

102. Which of the following best describes the author's intent in the passage?
    a. To entertain
    b. To inform
    c. To alert
    d. To suggest

103. Which of the following can be logically inferred from the passage?
    a. The Vikings disliked exploring the New World.
    b. Leif Erikson's banishment from Iceland led to his exploration of present-day Canada.
    c. Leif Erikson never shared his stories of exploration with the King of Norway.
    d. Historians have difficulty definitively pinpointing events in the Vikings' history.

Questions 104-117 are based on the following two passages:

Passage 1

Shakespeare and His Plays

People who argue that William Shakespeare is not responsible for the plays attributed to his name are known as anti-Stratfordians (from the name of Shakespeare's birthplace, Stratford-upon-Avon). The most common anti-Stratfordian claim is that William Shakespeare simply was not educated enough or from a high enough social class to have written plays overflowing with references to such a wide range of subjects like history, the classics, religion, and international culture. William Shakespeare was the son of a glove-maker, he only had a basic grade school education, and he never set foot outside of England—so how could he have produced plays of such sophistication and imagination? How could he have written in such detail about historical figures and events, or about different cultures and locations around Europe? According to anti-Stratfordians, the depth of knowledge contained in Shakespeare's plays suggests a well-traveled writer from a wealthy background with a university education, not a countryside writer like Shakespeare. But in fact, there is not much substance to such speculation, and most anti-Stratfordian arguments can be refuted with a little background about Shakespeare's time and upbringing.

First of all, those who doubt Shakespeare's authorship often point to his common birth and brief education as stumbling blocks to his writerly genius. Although it is true that Shakespeare did not come from a noble class, his father was a very *successful* glove-maker and his mother was from a very wealthy land-owning family—so while Shakespeare may have had a country upbringing, he was certainly from a well-off family and would have been educated accordingly. Also, even though he did not attend university, grade school education in Shakespeare's time was actually quite rigorous and exposed students to classic drama through writers like Seneca and Ovid. It is not unreasonable to believe that Shakespeare received a very solid foundation in poetry and literature from his early schooling.

Next, anti-Stratfordians tend to question how Shakespeare could write so extensively about countries and cultures he had never visited before (for instance, several of his most famous works like *Romeo and Juliet* and *The Merchant of Venice* were set in Italy, on the opposite side of Europe!). But again, this criticism does not hold up under scrutiny. For one thing, Shakespeare was living in London, a bustling metropolis of international trade, the most populous city in England, and a political and cultural hub of Europe. In the daily crowds of people, Shakespeare would certainly have been able to meet travelers from other countries and hear firsthand accounts of life in their home country. And, in addition to the influx of information from world travelers, this was also the age of the printing press, a jump in technology that made it possible to print and circulate books much more easily than in the past. This also allowed for a freer flow of information across different countries, allowing people to read about life and ideas from throughout Europe. One needn't travel the continent in order to learn and write about its culture.

Passage 2

The following passage is from The Shakespeare Problem Restated *by G.G. Greenwood*

Now there is very good authority for saying, and I think the truth is so, that at least two of the plays published among the works of Shakespeare are not his at all; that at least three others contain very little, if any, of his writing; and that of the remainder, many contain long passages that are non-Shakespearean. But when we have submitted them all the crucible of criticism we have a magnificent residuum of the purest gold. Here is the true Shakespeare; here is the great magician who, by a wave of his wand, could transmute brass into gold, or make dry bones live and move and have immortal being. Who was this great magician—this mighty dramatist who was "not of an age, but for all time"? Who was the writer of *Venus* and *Lucrece* and the *Sonnets* and *Lear* and *Hamlet*? Was it William Shakespeare of Stratford, the Player? So it is generally believed, and that hypothesis I had accepted in unquestioning faith till my love of the works naturally led me to an examination of the life of the supposed author of them. Then I found that as I read my faith melted away "into thin air." It was not, certainly, that I had (nor have I now) any wish to disbelieve. I was, and I am, altogether willing to accept the Player as the immortal poet if only my reason would allow me to do so. Why not? . . . But the question of authorship is, nevertheless, a most fascinating one. If it be true, as the Rev. Leonard Bacon wrote that "The great world does not care sixpence who wrote *Hamlet*," the great world must, at the same time, be a very small world, and many of us must be content to be outside it. Having given, then, the best attention I was able to give to the question, and more time, I fear, than I ought to have devoted to it, I was brought to the conclusion, as many others have been, that the man who is, truly enough, designated by Messrs. Garnett and Gosse as a "Stratford rustic" is not the true Shakespeare. . .

That Shakespeare the "Stratford rustic and London actor" should have acquired this learning, this culture, and this polish; that *he* should have travelled into foreign lands, studied the life and topography of foreign cities, and the manners and customs of all sorts and conditions of men; that *he* should have written some half-dozen dramas . . . besides qualifying himself as a professional actor; that *he* should have done all this and a good deal more between 1587 and 1592 is a supposition so wild that it can only be entertained by those who are prepared to accept it as a miracle. "And miracles do not happen!"

104. Which sentence contains the author's thesis in the first passage?
    a. People who argue that William Shakespeare is not responsible for the plays attributed to his name are known as anti-Stratfordians.
    b. But in fact, there is not much substance to such speculation, and most anti-Stratfordian arguments can be refuted with a little background about Shakespeare's time and upbringing.
    c. It is not unreasonable to believe that Shakespeare received a very solid foundation in poetry and literature from his early schooling.
    d. Next, anti-Stratfordians tend to question how Shakespeare could write so extensively about countries and cultures he had never visited before.

105. In the first paragraph in Passage 1, "How could he have written in such detail about historical figures and events, or about different cultures and locations around Europe?" is an example of which of the following?
    a. Hyperbole
    b. Onomatopoeia
    c. Rhetorical question
    d. Appeal to authority

106. In Passage 1, how does the author respond to the claim that Shakespeare was not well-educated because he did not attend university?
    a. By insisting upon Shakespeare's natural genius.
    b. By explaining grade school curriculum in Shakespeare's time.
    c. By comparing Shakespeare with other uneducated writers of his time.
    d. By pointing out that Shakespeare's wealthy parents probably paid for private tutors.

107. In Passage 1, the word *bustling* in the third paragraph most nearly means which of the following?
    a. Busy
    b. Foreign
    c. Expensive
    d. Undeveloped

108. In passage 2, the following sentence is an example of what?

    "Here is the true Shakespeare; here is the great magician who, by a wave of his wand, could transmute brass into gold, or make dry bones live and move and have immortal being."

    a. Personification
    b. Metaphor
    c. Simile
    d. Allusion

109. In passage 2, the author's attitude toward Stratfordians can be described as which of the following?
    a. Accepting and forgiving
    b. Uncaring and neutral
    c. Uplifting and admiring
    d. Disbelieving and critical

110. What is the relationship between these two sentences from Passage 2?

Sentence 1: So it is generally believed, and that hypothesis I had accepted in unquestioning faith till my love of the works naturally led me to an examination of the life of the supposed author of them.

Sentence 2: Then I found that as I read my faith melted away "into thin air."

a. Sentence 2 explains the main idea in Sentence 1.
b. Sentence 2 continues the definition begun in Sentence 1.
c. Sentence 2 analyzes the comment in Sentence 1.
d. Sentence 2 is a contrast to the idea in Sentence 1.

111. The writing style of Passage 1 could be best described as what?
a. Expository
b. Persuasive
c. Narrative
d. Descriptive

112. In passage 2, the word *topography* in the second paragraph most nearly means which of the following?
a. Climate features of an area.
b. Agriculture specific to place.
c. Shape and features of the Earth.
d. Aspects of humans within society.

113. The authors of the passages differ in their opinion of Shakespeare in that the author of Passage 2
a. Believes that Shakespeare the actor did not write the plays.
b. Believes that Shakespeare the playwright did not in act in the plays.
c. Believes that Shakespeare was both the actor and the playwright.
d. Believes that Shakespeare was neither the actor nor the playwright.

114. Which of the following would the two authors be most likely to disagree over?
a. Readers of Shakespeare's plays should not care whether or not the "country Shakespeare" wrote the plays or not; the fact that they exist is reason enough for readers to be grateful.
b. A person born into a lower socioeconomic class is not capable of writing plays with universal themes that creates new ways to use the English language.
c. That a country education is not sufficient enough to have written the greatest plays in Western Civilization.
d. That in order to write about the topography and civilization of a place, one must have travelled there and mingled with the people.

115. The author of Passage 1 believes that Shakespeare the actor *was* Shakespeare the writer because of which of the following?
   a. New evidence cites that Shakespeare did indeed travel a great bit between the years 1587 and 1592, suggesting that the playwright did have sufficient experience to write the great plays.
   b. There is sufficient evidence from Shakespeare's peers that proves that Shakespeare wrote the poems and plays that his name was signed to.
   c. An individual with Shakespeare's socioeconomic status and country education would be too limited in knowledge to write such brilliant plays.
   d. A country education and socioeconomic status do not deflect true genius if the individual is willing to absorb the textual and cultural knowledge surrounding them.

116. Which one of the following most accurately shows the relationship between the two passages?
   a. Passage 1 is written in concession with Passage 2.
   b. Passage 1 is written in opposition to Passage 2.
   c. Passage 1 is neutral to the stance of Passage 2.
   d. Passage 1 uses direct quotation from Passage 2 for contradiction.

117. The last phrase in this sentence in Passage 1 is considered what?

   William Shakespeare was the son of a glove-maker, he only had a basic grade school education, and he never set foot outside of England—so how could he have produced plays of such sophistication and imagination?

   a. Rhetorical question
   b. Literary allusion
   c. Hyperbole
   d. Symbolism

In this excerpt from a novel set in nineteenth-century France, two friends, Albert de Morcef and the Count of Monte Cristo, discuss Parisian social life. Read it and answer questions 118-124.

   "Mademoiselle Eugénie is pretty—I think I remember that to be her name."

   "Very pretty, or rather, very beautiful," replied Albert, "but of that style of beauty which I don't appreciate; I am an ungrateful fellow."

   "Really," said Monte Cristo, lowering his voice, "you don't appear to me to be very enthusiastic on the subject of this marriage."

   "Mademoiselle Danglars is too rich for me," replied Morcerf, "and that frightens me."

   "Bah," exclaimed Monte Cristo, "that's a fine reason to give. Are you not rich yourself?"

   "My father's income is about 50,000 francs per annum; and he will give me, perhaps, ten or twelve thousand when I marry."

   "That, perhaps, might not be considered a large sum, in Paris especially," said the count; "but everything doesn't depend on wealth, and it's a fine thing to have a good name, and to occupy a high station in society. Your name is celebrated, your position magnificent; and then the Comte de Morcerf is a soldier, and it's pleasing to see the integrity of a Bayard united to the poverty of a Duguesclin; disinterestedness is the brightest ray in which a noble sword can shine. As for me, I consider the union with Mademoiselle Danglars a most suitable one; she will enrich you, and you will ennoble her."

Albert shook his head, and looked thoughtful. "There is still something else," said he.

"I confess," observed Monte Cristo, "that I have some difficulty in comprehending your objection to a young lady who is both rich and beautiful."

"Oh," said Morcerf, "this repugnance, if repugnance it may be called, isn't all on my side."

"Whence can it arise, then? for you told me your father desired the marriage."

"It's my mother who dissents; she has a clear and penetrating judgment, and doesn't smile on the proposed union. I cannot account for it, but she seems to entertain some prejudice against the Danglars."

"Ah," said the count, in a somewhat forced tone, "that may be easily explained; the Comtesse de Morcerf, who is aristocracy and refinement itself, doesn't relish the idea of being allied by your marriage with one of ignoble birth; that is natural enough."

118. The meaning of the word "repugnance" is closest to:
    a. Strong resemblance
    b. Strong dislike
    c. Extreme shyness
    d. Extreme dissimilarity

119. What can be inferred about Albert's family?
    a. Their finances are uncertain.
    b. Albert is the only son in his family.
    c. Their name is more respected than the Danglars'.
    d. Albert's mother and father both agree on their decisions.

120. What is Albert's attitude towards his impending marriage?
    a. Pragmatic
    b. Romantic
    c. Indifferent
    d. Apprehensive

121. What is the best description of the Count's relationship with Albert?
    a. He's like a strict parent, criticizing Albert's choices.
    b. He's like a wise uncle, giving practical advice to Albert.
    c. He's like a close friend, supporting all of Albert's opinions.
    d. He's like a suspicious investigator, asking many probing questions.

122. Which sentence is true of Albert's mother?
    a. She belongs to a noble family.
    b. She often makes poor choices.
    c. She is primarily occupied with money.
    d. She is unconcerned about her son's future.

123. Based on this passage, what is probably NOT true about French society in the 1800s?
   a. Children often received money from their parents.
   b. Marriages were sometimes arranged between families.
   c. The richest people in society were also the most respected.
   d. People were often expected to marry within their same social class.

124. Why is the Count puzzled by Albert's attitude toward his marriage?
   a. He seems reluctant to marry Eugénie, despite her wealth and beauty.
   b. He is marrying against his father's wishes, despite usually following his advice.
   c. He appears excited to marry someone he doesn't love, despite being a hopeless romantic.
   d. He expresses reverence towards Eugénie, despite being from a higher social class than her.

A traveler prepares for a journey in this excerpt from a novel. Read it and answer questions 125-130.

When I got on the coach the driver had not taken his seat, and I saw him talking with the landlady. They were evidently talking of me, for every now and then they looked at me, and some of the people who were sitting on the bench outside the door came and listened, and then looked at me, most of them pityingly. I could hear a lot of words often repeated, queer words, for there were many nationalities in the crowd; so I quietly got my polyglot dictionary from my bag and looked them out. I must say they weren't cheering to me, for amongst them were "Ordog"—Satan, "pokol"—hell, "stregoica"—witch, "vrolok" and "vlkoslak"—both of which mean the same thing, one being Slovak and the other Servian for something that is either were-wolf or vampire.

When we started, the crowd round the inn door, which had by this time swelled to a considerable size, all made the sign of the cross and pointed two fingers towards me. With some difficulty I got a fellow-passenger to tell me what they meant; he wouldn't answer at first, but on learning that I was English, he explained that it was a charm or guard against the evil eye. This was not very pleasant for me, just starting for an unknown place to meet an unknown man; but everyone seemed so kind-hearted, and so sorrowful, and so sympathetic that I couldn't but be touched. I shall never forget the last glimpse which I had of the inn-yard and its crowd of picturesque figures, all crossing themselves, as they stood round the wide archway, with its background of rich foliage of oleander and orange trees in green tubs clustered in the centre of the yard. Then our driver cracked his big whip over his four small horses, which ran abreast, and we set off on our journey.

I soon lost sight and recollection of ghostly fears in the beauty of the scene as we drove along, although had I known the language, or rather languages, which my fellow-passengers were speaking, I might not have been able to throw them off so easily. Before us lay a green sloping land full of forests and woods, with here and there steep hills, crowned with clumps of trees or with farmhouses, the blank gable end to the road. There was everywhere a bewildering mass of fruit blossom—apple, plum, pear, cherry; and as we drove by I could see the green grass under the trees spangled with the fallen petals. In and out amongst these green hills of what they call here the "Mittel Land" ran the road, losing itself as it swept round the grassy curve, or was shut out by the straggling ends of pine woods, which here and there ran down the hillsides like tongues of flame. The road was rugged, but still we seemed to fly over it with a feverish haste. I couldn't understand then what the haste meant, but the driver was evidently bent on losing no time in reaching Borgo Prund.

125. What type of narrator is found in this passage?
   a. First person
   b. Second person
   c. Third-person limited
   d. Third-person omniscient

126. Which of the following is true of the traveler?
   a. He wishes the driver would go faster.
   b. He's returning to the country of his birth.
   c. He has some familiarity with the local customs.
   d. He doesn't understand all of the languages being used.

127. How does the traveler's mood change between the second and third paragraphs?
   a. From relaxed to rushed
   b. From fearful to charmed
   c. From confused to enlightened
   d. From comfortable to exhausted

128. Who is the traveler going to meet?
   a. A kind landlady
   b. A distant relative
   c. A friendly villager
   d. A complete stranger

129. Based on the details in this passage, what can readers probably expect to happen in the story?
   a. The traveler will become a farmer.
   b. The traveler will arrive late at his destination.
   c. The traveler will soon encounter danger or evil.
   d. The traveler will have a pleasant journey and make many new friends.

130. Which sentence from the passage provides a clue for question 39?
   a. "I must say they weren't cheering to me, for amongst them were "Ordog"—Satan, "pokol"—hell, "stregoica"—witch, "vrolok" and "vlkoslak"—both of which mean the same thing, one being Slovak and the other Servian for something that is either were-wolf or vampire."
   b. "When I got on the coach the driver had not taken his seat, and I saw him talking with the landlady."
   c. "Then our driver cracked his big whip over his four small horses, which ran abreast, and we set off on our journey."
   d. "There was everywhere a bewildering mass of fruit blossom—apple, plum, pear, cherry; and as we drove by I could see the green grass under the trees spangled with the fallen petals."

Questions 131 – 134 are based on the following passage.

Smoking tobacco products is terribly destructive. A single cigarette contains over 4,000 chemicals, including 43 known carcinogens and 400 deadly toxins. Some of the most dangerous ingredients include tar, carbon monoxide, formaldehyde, ammonia, arsenic, and DDT. Smoking can cause numerous types of cancer including throat, mouth, nasal cavity, esophagus, stomach, pancreas, kidney, bladder, and cervical.

Cigarettes contain a drug called nicotine, one of the most addictive substances known to man. Addiction is defined as a compulsion to seek the substance despite negative consequences. According to the National Institute of Drug Abuse, nearly 35 million smokers expressed a desire to quit smoking in 2015; however, more than 85 percent of those addicts will not achieve their goal. Almost all smokers regret picking up that first cigarette. You would be wise to learn from their mistake if you have not yet started smoking.

According to the U.S. Department of Health and Human Services, 16 million people in the United States presently suffer from a smoking-related condition and nearly nine million suffer from a serious smoking-related illness. According to the Centers for Disease Control and Prevention (CDC), tobacco products cause nearly six million deaths per year. This number is projected to rise to over eight million deaths by 2030. Smokers, on average, die ten years earlier than their nonsmoking peers.

In the United States, local, state, and federal governments typically tax tobacco products, which leads to high prices. Nicotine addicts sometimes pay more for a pack of cigarettes than for a few gallons of gas. Additionally, smokers tend to stink. The smell of smoke is all-consuming and creates a pervasive nastiness. Smokers also risk staining their teeth and fingers with yellow residue from the tar.

Smoking is deadly, expensive, and socially unappealing. Clearly, smoking is not worth the risks.

131. Which of the following best describes the passage?
    a. Narrative
    b. Persuasive
    c. Expository
    d. Technical

132. Which of the following statements most accurately summarizes the passage?
    a. Tobacco is less healthy than many alternatives.
    b. Tobacco is deadly, expensive, and socially unappealing, and smokers would be much better off kicking the addiction.
    c. In the United States, local, state, and federal governments typically tax tobacco products, which leads to high prices.
    d. Tobacco products shorten smokers' lives by ten years and kill more than six million people per year.

133. The author would be most likely to agree with which of the following statements?
    a. Smokers should only quit cold turkey and avoid all nicotine cessation devices.
    b. Other substances are more addictive than tobacco.
    c. Smokers should quit for whatever reason that gets them to stop smoking.
    d. People who want to continue smoking should advocate for a reduction in tobacco product taxes.

134. Which of the following represents an opinion statement on the part of the author?
    a. According to the Centers for Disease Control and Prevention (CDC), tobacco products cause nearly six million deaths per year.
    b. Nicotine addicts sometimes pay more for a pack of cigarettes than a few gallons of gas.
    c. They also risk staining their teeth and fingers with yellow residue from the tar.
    d. Additionally, smokers tend to stink. The smell of smoke is all-consuming and creates a pervasive nastiness.

The following passage is an excerpt from Civil Disobedience, *by Henry David Thoreau. Please read it and answer questions 135 – 140.*

I heartily accept the motto, "that government is best which governs least," and I should like to see it acted up to more rapidly and systematically. Carried out, it finally amounts to this, which also I believe—"that government is best which governs not at all," and when men are prepared for it, that will be the kind of government which they will have. Government is at best but an expedient; but most governments are usually, and all governments are sometimes, inexpedient. The objections which have been brought against a standing army, and they are many and weighty, and deserve to prevail, may also at last be brought against a standing government. The standing army is only an arm of the standing government. The government itself, which is only the mode which the people have chosen to execute their will, is equally liable to be abused and perverted before the people can act through it. Witness the present Mexican war, the work of comparatively a few individuals using the standing government as their tool; for, in the outset, the people would not have consented to this measure.

This American government—what is it but a tradition, though a recent one, endeavoring to transmit itself unimpaired to posterity, but each instant losing some of its integrity? It has not the vitality and force of a single living man; for a single man can bend it to his will. It is a sort of wooden gun to the people themselves. But it is not the less necessary for this; for the people must have some complicated machinery or other, and hear its din, to satisfy that idea of government which they have. Governments show thus how successfully men can be imposed on, even impose on themselves, for their own advantage. It is excellent, we must all allow. Yet this government never of itself furthered any enterprise, but by the alacrity with which it got out of its way. It does not keep the country free. It does not settle the West. It does not educate. The character inherent in the American people has done all that has been accomplished; and it would have done somewhat more, if the government had not sometimes got in its way. For government is an expedient by which men would fain succeed in letting one another alone; and, as has been said, when it is most expedient, the governed are most let alone by it. Trade and commerce, if they were not made of india-rubber, would never manage to bounce over the obstacles which legislators are continually putting in their way; and, if one were to judge these men wholly by the effects of their actions and not partly by their intentions, they would deserve to be classed and punished with those mischievous persons who put obstructions on the railroads.

But, to speak practically and as a citizen, unlike those who call themselves no-government men, I ask for, not at once no government, but at once a better government. Let every man make known what kind of government would command his respect, and that will be one step toward obtaining it.

135. Which phrase best encapsulates Thoreau's use of the term *expedient* in the first paragraph?
    a. A dead end
    b. A state of order
    c. A means to an end
    d. Rushed construction

136. Which best describes Thoreau's view on the Mexican War?
    a. Government is inherently corrupt because it must wage war.
    b. Government can easily be manipulated by a few individuals for their own agenda.
    c. Government is a tool for the people, but it can also act against their interest.
    d. The Mexican War was a necessary action, but not all the people believed this.

137. What is Thoreau's purpose for writing?
    a. His goal is to illustrate how government can function if ideals are maintained.
    b. He wants to prove that true democracy is the best government, but it can be corrupted easily.
    c. Thoreau reflects on the stages of government abuses.
    d. He is seeking to prove that government is easily corruptible and inherently restrictive of individual freedoms that can simultaneously affect the whole state.

138. Which example best supports Thoreau's argument?
    a. A vote carries in the Senate to create a new road tax.
    b. The president vetoes the new FARM bill.
    c. Prohibition is passed to outlaw alcohol.
    d. Trade is opened between the United States and Iceland.

139. Which best summarizes this section from the following passage?
    "This American government—what is it but a tradition, though a recent one, endeavoring to transmit itself unimpaired to posterity, but each instant losing some of its integrity? It has not the vitality and force of a single living man; for a single man can bend it to his will. It is a sort of wooden gun to the people themselves."

    a. The government may be instituted to ensure the protections of freedoms, but this is weakened by the fact that it is easily manipulated by individuals.
    b. Unlike an individual, government is uncaring.
    c. Unlike an individual, government has no will, making it more prone to be used as a weapon against the people.
    d. American government is modeled after other traditions but actually has greater potential to be used to control people.

140. According to Thoreau, what's the main reason why government eventually fails to achieve progress?
    a. There are too many rules.
    b. Legislation eventually becomes a hindrance to the lives and work of everyday people.
    c. Trade and wealth eventually become the driving factor of those in government.
    d. Government doesn't separate religion and state.

The following passage is an excerpt from "Contributions to the Energetics of Evolution," by Alfred J. Lotka. Please read this and answer questions 141 – 146.

It has been pointed out by Boltzmann that the fundamental object of contention in the life-struggle, in the evolution of the organic world, is available energy. In accord with this observation is the principle that, in the struggle for existence, the advantage must go to those organisms whose energy-capturing devices are most efficient in directing available energy into channels favorable to the preservation of the species.

The first effect of natural selection thus operating upon competing species will be to give relative preponderance (in number or mass) to those most efficient in guiding available energy in the manner indicated. Primarily the path of the energy flux through the system will be affected.

But the species possessing superior energy-capturing and directing devices may accomplish something more than merely to divert to its own advantage energy for which others are competing with it. If sources are presented, capable of supplying available energy in excess of that actually being tapped by the entire system of living organisms, then an opportunity is furnished for suitably constituted organisms to enlarge the total energy flux through the system. Whenever such organisms arise, natural selection will operate to preserve and increase them. The result, in this case, is not a mere diversion of the energy flux through the system of organic nature along a new path, but an increase of the total flux through that system.

Again, so long as sources exist, capable of supplying matter, of a character suitable for the composition of living organisms, in excess of that actually embodied in the system of organic nature, so long is opportunity furnished for suitably constituted organisms to enlarge the total mass of the system of organic nature. Whenever such organisms arise, natural selection will operate to preserve and increase them, provided always that there is presented a residue of untapped available energy. The result will be to increase the total mass of the system, and, with this total mass, also the total energy flux through the system, since, other things equal, this energy flux is proportional to the mass of the system.

Where a limit, either constant or slowly changing, is imposed upon the total mass available for the operation of life processes, the available energy per unit of time (available power) placed at the disposal of the organisms, for application to their life tasks and contests, may be capable of increase by increasing the rate of turnover of the organic matter through the life cycle. So, for example, under present conditions, the United States produces annually a crop of primary and secondary food amounting to about 1.37×10^{14} kilogram-calories per annum, enough to support a population of about 105 million persons (equivalent to about 88 million adults) at the present rate of food consumption (4,270 kilogram-calories per adult per day). Suppose, as a simple, though rather extreme illustration, that man found means of doubling the rate of growth of crops, and of growing two crops a year instead of one. Then, without changing the average crop actually standing on the fields, the land would be capable of supporting double the present population. If this population were attained, the energy flux through the system composed of the human population and the organisms upon which it is dependent for food would also be doubled. This result would be attained, not by doubling the mass of the system (for the matter locked up in crops, etc., at a given moment would be, on an average, unchanged) but by increasing the velocity of circulation of mass through the life cycle in the system. Once more it is evident that, whenever a group of organisms arises which is so constituted as to increase the rate of circulation of matter through the system in the manner exemplified, natural selection will operate to preserve and increase such a group, provided always that there is presented a residue of untapped available energy—and, where circumstances require it, also a residue of mass suitable for the composition of living matter.

141. Judging by the content of the passage, Boltzmann (opening paragraph) is most likely which of the following?
  a. Physicist
  b. Dietician
  c. Anthropologist
  d. Agriculturalist

142. Which description best suits the use of "competing" in the first line of the second paragraph?
  a. Varying in diversity
  b. Fighting to the death
  c. Coexisting in the land
  d. Seeking to develop

143. What is the author's purpose behind writing this passage?
  a. To educate the reader on how energy conservation impacts genetic development
  b. To disprove the idea that energy is not essential to evolution
  c. To advocate the study of environmental enhancements to increase resource availability
  d. To prove that an organism's ability to capture and retain energy influences its survival and evolution

144. It would be reasonable to assume that a "species possessing superior energy-capturing and directing devices" would do which of the following?
  a. Die out from having too much energy
  b. Thrive and pass on these energy-directing devices to the next generation
  c. Be unable to pass on these specific traits
  d. Disrupt the flux of the natural world

145. Which is the best correlation among energy, mass, and evolution?
  a. Energy creates evolutionary trends that result in shifting mass amounts.
  b. In the end, evolution is influenced by, but not dependent on, the mass and energy consumed by organisms.
  c. More mass means more energy, which makes evolution happen faster.
  d. The amount of energy consumed by organisms influences the total mass of their system, in turn, evolving energy-retaining traits.

146. Which phrase provides another example for what the author talks about in the following section of the passage?
  "This result would be attained, not by doubling the mass of the system (for the matter locked up in crops, etc., at a given moment would be, on an average, unchanged) but by increasing the velocity of circulation of mass through the life cycle in the system."

  a. Increasing a battery's mass enables it to store more power.
  b. If a treadmill is set to consistently turn for an hour, it produces double its own worth of electrical current.
  c. The stream that turns a wheel mill doesn't grow significantly after a storm but picks up significant speed, resulting in more power being generated by the mill.
  d. By building three windmills, wind power is tripled for a house.

The following excerpt is from the article "The Lancashire Witches 1612–2012," by Robert Poole. Please read it and answer questions 147 – 152.

Four hundred years ago, in 1612, the north-west of England was the scene of England's biggest peacetime witch trial: the trial of the Lancashire witches. Twenty people, mostly from the Pendle area of Lancashire, were imprisoned in the castle as witches. Ten were hanged, one died in gaol, one was sentenced to stand in the pillory, and eight were acquitted. The 2012 anniversary sees a small flood of commemorative events, including works of fiction by Blake Morrison, Carol Ann Duffy, and Jeanette Winterson. How did this witch trial come about, and what accounts for its enduring fame?

We know so much about the Lancashire Witches because the trial was recorded in unique detail by the clerk of the court, Thomas Potts, who published his account soon afterwards as *The Wonderful Discovery of Witches in the County of Lancaster*. I have recently published a modern-English edition of this book, together with an essay piecing together what we know of the events of 1612. It has been a fascinating exercise, revealing how Potts carefully edited the evidence, and also how the case against the "witches" was constructed and manipulated to bring about a spectacular show trial. It all began in mid-March when a pedlar from Halifax named John Law had a frightening encounter with a poor young woman, Alizon Device, in a field near Colne. He refused her request for pins and there was a brief argument during which he was seized by a fit that left him with "his head … drawn awry, his eyes and face deformed, his speech not well to be understood; his thighs and legs stark lame." We can now recognize this as a stroke, perhaps triggered by the stressful encounter. Alizon Device was sent for and surprised all by confessing to the bewitching of John Law and then begged for forgiveness.

When Alizon Device was unable to cure the pedlar, the local magistrate, Roger Nowell was called in. Characterized by Thomas Potts as "God's justice" he was alert to instances of witchcraft, which were regarded by the Lancashire's puritan-inclined authorities as part of the cultural rubble of "popery"—Roman Catholicism—long overdue to be swept away at the end of the county's very slow protestant reformation. "With weeping tears" Alizon explained that she had been led astray by her grandmother, "old Demdike," well-known in the district for her knowledge of old Catholic prayers, charms, cures, magic, and curses. Nowell quickly interviewed Alizon's grandmother and mother, as well as Demdike's supposed rival, "old Chattox" and her daughter Anne. Their panicky attempts to explain themselves and shift the blame to others eventually only ended up incriminating them, and the four were sent to Lancaster gaol in early April to await trial at the summer assizes. The initial picture revealed was of a couple of poor, marginal local families in the forest of Pendle with a longstanding reputation for magical powers, which they had occasionally used at the request of their wealthier neighbours. There had been disputes but none of these were part of ordinary village life. Not until 1612 did any of this come to the attention of the authorities.

The net was widened still further at the end of April when Alizon's younger brother James and younger sister Jennet, only nine years old, came up between them with a story about a "great meeting of witches" at their grandmother's house, known as Malkin Tower. This meeting was presumably to discuss the plight of those arrested and the threat of further arrests, but according to the evidence extracted from the children by the magistrates, a plot was hatched to blow up Lancaster castle with gunpowder, kill the gaoler, and rescue the imprisoned witches. It was, in short, a conspiracy against royal authority to rival the gunpowder plot of 1605—

something to be expected in a county known for its particularly strong underground Roman Catholic presence.

Those present at the meeting were mostly family members and neighbours, but they also included Alice Nutter, described by Potts as "a rich woman [who] had a great estate, and children of good hope: in the common opinion of the world, of good temper, free from envy or malice." Her part in the affair remains mysterious, but she seems to have had Catholic family connections, and may have been one herself, providing an added motive for her to be prosecuted.

147. What's the point of this passage, and why did the author write it?
    a. The author is documenting a historic witchcraft trial while uncovering/investigating the role of suspicion and anti-Catholicism in the events.
    b. The author seeks long-overdue reparations for the ancestors of those accused and executed for witchcraft in Lancashire.
    c. The author is educating the reader about actual occult practices of the 1600s.
    d. The author argues that the Lancashire witch trials were more brutal than the infamous Salem trials.

148. Which term best captures the meaning of the author's use of "enduring" in the first paragraph?
    a. Un-original
    b. Popular
    c. Wicked
    d. Circumstantial

149. What textual information is present within the passage that most lends itself to the author's credibility?
    a. His prose is consistent with the time.
    b. This is a reflective passage; the author doesn't need to establish credibility.
    c. The author cites specific quotes.
    d. The author has published a modern account of the case and has written on the subject before.

150. What might the following excerpt suggest about the trial or, at the very least, Thomas Potts' account of the trial(s)?
    "It has been a fascinating exercise, revealing how Potts carefully edited the evidence, and also how the case against the 'witches' was constructed and manipulated to bring about a spectacular show trial."

    a. The events were so grand that the public was allowed access to such a spectacular set of cases.
    b. Sections may have been exaggerated or stretched to create notoriety on an extraordinary case.
    c. Evidence was faked, making the trial a total farce.
    d. The trial was corrupt from the beginning.

151. Which statement best describes the political atmosphere of the 1600s that influenced the Alizon Device witch trial/case?

    a. Fear of witches was prevalent during this period.

    b. Magistrates were seeking ways to cement their power during this period of unrest.

    c. In a highly superstitious culture, the Protestant church and government were highly motivated to root out any potential sources that could undermine the current regime.

    d. Lancashire was originally a prominent area for pagan celebration, making the modern Protestants very weary of whispers of witchcraft and open to witch trials to resolve any potential threats to Christianity.

152. Which best describes the strongest "evidence" used in the case against Alizon and the witches?

    a. Knowledge of the occult and witchcraft

    b. "Spectral evidence"

    c. Popular rumors of witchcraft and Catholic association

    d. Self-incriminating speech

The following passage is an excerpt from The Myth of the Birth of the Hero, A Psychological Interpretation of Mythology, *by Otto Rank. Read it and answer questions 153 – 158.*

> The prominent civilized nations—the Babylonians and Egyptians, the Hebrews and Hindus, the Persians, the Greeks and the Romans, as well as the Teutons and others—all began at an early stage to glorify their national heroes—mythical princes and kings, founders of religions, dynasties, empires, or cities—in a number of poetic tales and legends. The history of the birth and of the early life of these personalities came to be especially invested with fantastic features, which in different nations—even though widely separated by space and entirely independent of each other—present a baffling similarity or, in part, a literal correspondence. Many investigators have long been impressed with this fact, and one of the chief problems of mythological research still consists in the elucidation of the reason for the extensive analogies in the fundamental outlines of mythical tales, which are rendered still more puzzling by the unanimity in certain details and their reappearance in most of the mythical groupings.

> The mythological theories, aiming at the explanation of these remarkable phenomena, are, in a general way, as follows:

> 1. The "Idea of the People," propounded by Adolf Bastian. This theory assumes the existence of elemental ideas, so that the unanimity of the myths is a necessary sequence of the uniform disposition of the human mind and the manner of its manifestation, which within certain limits is identical at all times and in all places. This interpretation was urgently advocated by Adolf Bauer as accounting for the wide distribution of the hero myths.

> 2. The explanation by original community, first applied by Theodor Benfey to the widely distributed parallel forms of folklore and fairy tales. Originating in a favorable locality (India), these tales were first accepted by the primarily related (Indo-Germanic) peoples, then continued to grow while retaining the common primary traits, and ultimately radiated over the entire earth. This mode of explanation was first adapted to the wide distribution of the hero myths by Rudolf Schubert.

3. The modern theory of migration, or borrowing, according to which individual myths originate from definite peoples (especially the Babylonians) and are accepted by other peoples through oral tradition (commerce and traffic) or through literary influences. The modern theory of migration and borrowing can be readily shown to be merely a modification of Benfey's theory, necessitated by newly discovered and irreconcilable material. This profound and extensive research of modern investigations has shown that India, rather than Babylonia, may be regarded as the first home of the myths. Moreover, the tales presumably did not radiate from a single point, but traveled over and across the entire inhabited globe. This brings into prominence the idea of the interdependence of mythological structures, an idea which was generalized by Braun as the basic law of the nature of the human mind: Nothing new is ever discovered as long as it is possible to copy. The theory of elemental ideas, so strenuously advocated by Bauer over a quarter of a century ago, is unconditionally declined by the most recent investigators (Winckler, Stucken), who maintain the migration theory.

There is really no such sharp contrast between the various theories or their advocates, for the concept of elemental ideas does not interfere with the claims of primary common possession or of migration. Furthermore, the ultimate problem is not whence and how the material reached a certain people; the question is: Where did it come from to begin with? All these theories would explain only the variability and distribution of the myths, but not their origin. Even Schubert, the most inveterate opponent of Bauer's view, acknowledges this truth, by stating that all these manifold sagas date back to a single very ancient prototype. But he is unable to tell us anything of the origin of this prototype. Bauer likewise inclines to this mediating view; he points out repeatedly that in spite of the multiple origin of independent tales, it is necessary to concede a most extensive and ramified borrowing, as well as an original community of the concepts in related peoples.

153. Which term best defines *elucidation* as it's used in the first paragraph of the passage?
   a. Definition
   b. Specification
   c. Ramification
   d. Explanation

154. Based on the title of his work and the context of the selected passage, which statement may serve as the best explanation for why Rank is studying mythology?
   a. Psychologist Carl Jung proved the concept of archetypes seems to suggest universal concepts and ideas.
   b. The proliferation of common mythic structures around the world and cultures suggest shared, fundamental human ideas and values. To study these myths is to study the core of human thought.
   c. The study of the mythic hero may uncover the true origins of the first leaders.
   d. Studying mythology enables Rank to analyze how conflicts can be mitigated across various cultures, helping him develop new psychological analysis strategies and therapies.

155. Which statement provides an example that would correlate the following theory from the main passage?
   "The 'Idea of the People,' propounded by Adolf Bastian. This theory assumes the existence of elemental ideas, so that the unanimity of the myths is a necessary sequence of the uniform disposition of the human mind and the manner of its manifestation, which within certain limits is identical at all times and in all places."

a. Human beings have the need to understand their origins, hence the presence of creation myths.

b. The idea of winter as a cold season needed explanation; therefore, myths developed to analyze and interpret the natural phenomena, creating stories that account for seasonal change.

c. Heroes exemplify power and strength.

d. The Germanic and Nordic people wanted to understand why chaos exists in the world; the giants, beings of chaos and destruction, explained how natural phenomena occurred.

156. Reading through the body of the text, why is it appropriate that the mentioned theories are in fact called *theories*?

a. They are scientific explanations.

b. There is no reason; this was an artistic choice.

c. While very insightful, these theories as of yet cannot be officially proven; however, they are likely.

d. These are all competing ideas.

157. What are some insights that can be drawn from the following description of the third theory of mythic origins statement that can also relate to the rest of the passage?

"This brings into prominence the idea of the interdependence of mythological structures, an idea which was generalized by Braun as the basic law of the nature of the human mind: Nothing new is ever discovered as long as it is possible to copy."

a. Humans lack originality; there are no new ideas.

b. The cultural minds of human beings evolved from a set of basic ideas.

c. Human culture is interdependent on one another; there is no unique culture but a sundered mythic cycle that once was universal.

d. Recurring mythic structures seem to be reiterations of shared human experiences/stories, used over and over but modified throughout various cultures.

158. Which answer best exemplifies the mentioned theory/explanation in the following description of the second theory of mythic origins?

"The explanation by original community, first applied by Theodor Benfey to the widely distributed parallel forms of folklore and fairy tales. Originating in a favorable locality (India), these tales were first accepted by the primarily related (Indo-Germanic) peoples, then continued to grow while retaining the common primary traits, and ultimately radiated over the entire earth."

a. A tribe begins trading with another tribe. Through this interaction, different myths are shared, including the story of the hero.

b. A tribe has a legend of how the sky was formed. At some point, the tribe splits into different tribes, and each retains the myth. Some of the newer tribes attribute sky creation to different gods or tricksters.

c. The myth of Aeneas and Dido explains the ancient rivalry between Carthage and Rome.

d. There is a myth of a world flood in many cultures.

The following excerpt is from "The Culture Emergence of Man", by Alton Howard Thompson. Read it and answer questions 159 – 164.

Dr. Frank Baker, of the National Zoological Park, at Washington, kindly wrote that "One monkey in our collection, when annoyed by visitors, will throw anything, from a feed-pan to a handful of sawdust, at an offender. One Cebus tried to pick cockroaches out of the cracks in the floor with a straw, when too small for his fingers; but beyond this there has been nothing observed that could be considered as the using of an object as a tool or weapon." Other correspondents said the same thing—there were no actions on the part of the quadrumana, that they had observed, that could be taken as indicative of intelligent action. Prof. R. L. Garner, in his most interesting book on the "Speech of Apes and Monkeys," who spent some time in the wild country of the Gaboon on purpose to pursue his studies, observes that "animals may be taught to do many things in a mechanical way and without any motives that relate to the actions." His pet chimpanzee tried to drive nails, use the saw, etc., but could not manage it, nor even the use of the club to crush his sugar-cane. Of the gorilla he says: "As to his throwing sticks or stones at enemies, there is nothing to verify it and much to contradict it. It is a mere freak of fancy. Neither the chimpanzee nor the gorilla close the hand to strike nor use any weapon but the hands and teeth."

From this evidence at first hand, we must conclude that the use of extraneous substances by animals, especially the quadrumana, is purely automatic and imitative, and not to be considered as rational action at all. Whatever they have learned has been by reason of contact with man and the result of imitation and training. We must conclude, further, that the use of tools and weapons, even preceding the intelligent conformation of them for definite purposes, marked the differentiation of primitive man from the animal branch, and accompanied indeed was the cause of the psychic emergence. The moment that the primitive man-ape employed extraneous substances intelligently, with a purpose, he ceased to be an ape and became a man. We must believe that the use of tools and the psychic emergence were coincident and interdependent.

As M. de Pressense says, in his "Study of Origins" (352): "The first tool fashioned by man asserted his royalty over nature. Thus, the tool is man's true scepter; whether made of flint or wood or anything else—it is the result of thought. This is why the animal, guided by instinct, can affect marvels of construction by the use of its own limbs, but it never makes a tool. A monkey may have chanced one day to lean upon a stick, but he did not cut nor shape the stick nor hand it down to posterity, that they might improve upon it."

The struggles of the first ape-man to maintain life amid the hostile surroundings in which he found himself are fraught with peculiar interest, and are indeed almost pathetic when we consider the great odds that were against him in the fight. His natural weapons of defense, the jaws and teeth, were being reduced with a rapidity that must soon have brought about his extinction but for the correlative development of the grasping powers of the hand, which enabled him to employ and supplement his natural organs with the extra natural resources around him. And then it followed, as this grasping power enabled him to use a club or a stone, that some superior individual made a conscious effort to employ these weapons with more precision and initiate new purposes, and that he thereby learned to think. This was the divine spark that awakened mental life, which acted as a stimulus on the motor nerve centers, and these centers were enlarged by the effort to think. Then, as the brain grew, he could think more, and as he thought more his brain grew, and he became a man. If you will pardon the solecism, this primeval man might have said with Descartes (much to Descartes's surprise, probably, by the application), "Cogito; ergo sum"—I think; therefore I exist. It is an old and true saying that "man is the wisest of animals because of his hands"—a pre-Darwinian appreciation of correlated development that was prophetic.

We must begin, then, with the first efforts of primitive man to isolate himself from the animal world by the use of his hands, and the exercise of that manual power which distinguishes him from the rest of the animal kingdom and made him its master. We must consider, however, that primeval man was at first incapable of manufacturing implements and weapons from the materials around him, and was only capable of using in a simple way the gifts of nature as they came from her hands without any modification whatever. Kindly nature furnished him with these resources to supplement the waning powers of his natural organs, which were being rapidly modified in the process of his evolution. Primitive man utilized the simple things that nature furnished ready to his hand and they were sufficient for his needs. The primeval life of the human race must therefore be considered first in the light of what nature provided for practical use and which was of vital importance in the struggle for existence. But these were sufficient to give him the balance of power, and he lived. To this primeval man nature was kind and beneficent, and nursed and nurtured him to the full development of the maturity of the race, in his civilized descendants. From a mere animal she enabled him to develop into the godlike being who dominates the earth.

159. Which example of observation and/or discovery disproves the following excerpt from the passage? "From this evidence at first hand, we must conclude that the use of extraneous substances by animals, especially the quadrumana, is purely automatic and imitative, and not to be considered as rational action at all."

    a. Gorillas, chimpanzees, and orangutans have successfully learned sign language from humans.
    b. Modern chimpanzees have been discovered using stone tools in the wild.
    c. A Capuchin monkey learned to use a screwdriver for several advanced tasks after watching a video.
    d. Captive apes have taught their offspring sign language without being instructed by human trainers.

160. The term *quadrumana* is used multiple times in the text. What is the most accurate definition for this word that can be inferred from the text?
    a. Primates with four grasping hands
    b. Primates that evolved in the last forty thousand years
    c. Primates with five digits on each hand
    d. The classification of monkeys and great apes that spend time both in the trees and on the ground

161. What's the significance of the "psychic emergence" mentioned in the second paragraph?
    a. It represents the development of the frontal lobe, crucial for processing higher thoughts.
    b. It represents the development of mental powers needed to shape weapons.
    c. It represents the cognizance that items can be shaped and used for a purpose.
    d. It represents the development of free will.

162. Which answer best explains how Descartes' famous quote, "Cogito ergo sum," which Thompson translates to "I think; therefore, I exist," illustrates the author's main point?
    a. Being able to think is crucial to tool use.
    b. Self-awareness enables individuals to see nature objectively, so they will intentionally use resources and make decisions to advance their own existence.
    c. Self-awareness is what led to humans developing higher mental functions and tool making.
    d. The ability to understand natural resources and use was the beginning of the concept of individual thought and ambition to create.

163. Which best describes how the term *scepter* serves as an appropriate metaphor in Thompson's quote from M. de Pressense's *Study of Origins*, "Thus the tool is man's true scepter"?

    a. It symbolizes kingship and the ability to create and settle the world.

    b. It is a precious tool.

    c. It illustrates the inherited right for humans to rule the world due to their intelligence.

    d. It serves to illustrate man's independence and power to control natural elements (tools).

164. Which circumstance would the author argue is the most unlikely circumstance that could have contributed to "man-ape" developing the use of tools?

    a. Sleeping in caves provided shelter, so the apes consciously chose to seek caves.

    b. The presence of predators necessitated the use of objects to supplement the apes' defenses.

    c. Nutritious roots grow underground—realizing sticks are more proficient than arboreal fingernails, the apes started using sticks as digging tools.

    d. The apes struggled breaking into hard nuts; yet, discovering the weight and hardness of rocks, the apes began dropping rocks on the nuts to crack open the shells.

The following passage is from "The Rise of Natural History Museums," by Oliver Cummings Farrington. Please read it and answer questions 165 – 170.

A desire to preserve objects of nature which aroused special interest or possessed unusual powers may be presumed to have been an instinct of the earliest man. We may imagine the cave man storing in his cave the bright gem, or curious seed, or rare animal skin which attracted his attention and, perchance, urging upon his descendants the desirability of preserving it. Such instincts are undoubtedly possessed by barbarous tribes. But such hoards have no permanent value or maintenance as long as there is a lack of a fixed habitation or of a social organization sufficiently strong to pass them from one generation to another. Hence, it may be noted in passing, an essential condition for the existence of museums is a sufficiently civilized and permanent state of society to preserve objects from generation to generation.

In the life of the ancient Egyptians conditions making toward the preservation of natural objects doubtless became more favorable than had previously been the case, since there are preserved to us from their time many objects of their art which were originally objects of nature. While material which they prized now occupies an honored place in our museums and their civilization was instrumental in preserving it to us, there is no evidence, so far as I know, that they undertook the collection and preservation of natural objects for their own sake.

The Greeks gave us the word museum, but that they ever established a museum in the modern sense seems very unlikely. Whatever their practice may have been regarding the preservation and exhibition of works of art, it seems quite certain that they carried on little, if any, effort of this kind with regard to nature. Alexander the Great, about 325 BC, is said to have gathered together many animals and plants in order that they might be studied by Aristotle, "the father of natural history," but so far as we know no effort was made to preserve these specimens to later times. The first record of placing natural history specimens on exhibition is said to be made when Hanno, a Carthaginian, somewhat before Alexander's time, procured skins of gorillas in Africa and put them in the temple of Astarte. We also know that the monstrous horns of wild bulls which had occasioned great devastation in Macedonia were hung in the temple of Hercules by order of King Philip.

The Romans seem, like the Greeks, not to have taken much interest in the preservation of natural objects, at least as far as any record has reached the present time. We know that emperors and other individuals possessed collections of statues and other works of art, and among these we find occasional mention of the preservation of so-called "natural curiosities," such as bones of giants or peculiar human skeletons, but that any broad interest in nature existed which led to efforts to preserve and study its forms we have no record. Stray sources of information tell us of a crocodile, found in attempting to discover the sources of the Nile, being preserved in the temple of Isis at Cesarea, also that a large piece of the root of the cinnamon tree was kept in a golden vessel in one of the temples at Rome. Pliny relates that the bones of a sea monster, probably a whale, "to which Andromeda was exposed," were preserved at Joppa and afterwards brought to Rome. Suetonious says that the Emperor Augustus had a collection of natural curiosities in his palace.

One reason suggested by Beckmann for the rarity of collections of natural objects among ancient peoples was the lack of knowledge of satisfactory means of preserving such as were perishable. The preservative virtues of what was then called "spirit of wine," but which we now know as alcohol, seem to have been but little known, and only immersion in salt brine or a covering with wax or honey served at that time for the preservation of perishable materials.

The great institute of Alexandria in Egypt, founded in the third century BC, is generally spoken of as being the first natural-history museum of antiquity, but while this had botanical and zoological gardens, there is little reason to suppose that it was a museum of nature in the modern sense. The name museum in that institution was applied to a portion set apart for the study of sciences, and indicated rather a place of study than one for exhibition of objects.

165. Which statement best captures the goal of this excerpt?
    a. The author argues that the ancient Greeks, not the Egyptians, invented museums.
    b. The author is reflecting on the history of museums while detailing his own visits to museums.
    c. The author seeks to sketch the history behind modern museums by discussing ancient roots.
    d. The author wants to prove that actual museums didn't evolve until the 1850s.

166. Which best encapsulates the core reasoning behind the author's idea, "Hence, it may be noted in passing, an essential condition for the existence of museums is a sufficiently civilized and permanent state of society to preserve objects from generation to generation"?
    a. A refined level of sophistication is needed to understand and pass down the knowledge of artifacts within a museum.
    b. Stable civil conditions and a learned society are key for museum preservation and education; if the city is unstable, museum interest and artifacts are threatened.
    c. Museums can't exist as a nomadic, or traveling practice; the artifacts won't be preserved.
    d. The continuation of museums relies on educating future generations.

167. What seems to be the main criteria for a site to be considered a museum in the modern sense?
    a. A location that contain artifacts that are archaic in nature and significant to specific events
    b. A central location that houses artifacts
    c. The wealth to purchase items and display them safely without risk of damage or theft
    d. A central location that displays artifacts for the general public to learn and enjoy

168. Which of the following could best replace the term *virtues* in the fifth paragraph?
   a. Properties
   b. Corrections
   c. Understanding
   d. Abilities

169. What can be inferred from the following detail the author offers in the text?
   "Alexander the Great, about 325 BC, is said to have gathered together many animals and plants in order that they might be studied by Aristotle, 'the father of natural history,' but so far as we know no effort was made to preserve these specimens to later time."

   a. Aristotle was the best expert on natural history of his time.
   b. Collections like this led to the discovery of many exotic animals.
   c. Natural history and sciences were actively being studied in ancient times.
   d. Alexander the Great was seeking to build his own museum.

170. The author has decided to include a section that details how the "natural curiosities" that were often attributed to myths and legends were actually misidentified dinosaur bones, or other natural objects. Where would this information fit best?
   a. In a new paragraph, after the second paragraph
   b. In the fourth paragraph, before the last sentence
   c. Just above the last paragraph
   d. In the fourth paragraph, after the second sentence

The following passage is an excerpt from "Climatic Change and Agricultural Exhaustion as Elements in the Fall of Rome," by Ellsworth Huntington. Please read it and answer questions 171 – 176.

In history, as in science, the normal order is from obvious facts to hidden causes. The fact of the disastrous fall of Rome is so obvious that every intelligent person is aware of it. Its causes are so obscure that the world is still uncertain what they are. Among the many theories advanced in explanation of this great historical event, one of the most interesting is that of Liebig, which has recently been admirably restated by Professor Simkhovitch. According to the view of these two authors, one of the fundamental factors in the fall of Rome was a marked decline in agriculture. We are told that in the days of the Roman Republic seven jugera, or about four and one-half acres of land, sufficed for the tillage required to support an average family. Agriculture was so intensive that farms of this small size, supplemented presumably by pasture land, supported a contented, self-respecting, and progressive population. The cities, all of which were small, reflected the sturdy independence of the country people, and naturally the government was modeled to fit the citizens who administered it. By the second century before Christ, however, a great change was apparent. Under Scipio in 196 BC, grain began to be distributed from state granaries to poor citizens. Soon came the agrarian troubles with which the names of the Gracchi are associated. Seven jugera were no longer sufficient for the average farmer. Indeed, the farmers in many places were becoming poverty stricken. Instead of sowing their fields with a scientific rotation of carefully tilled crops, they were turning them over to pasturage. Cato declared that good pasturage was the best thing for a farmer, fair pasturage the second best, poor pasturage the third best, and ordinary field crops only the fourth resource. Pessimists declared that in their wheat fields the farmers reaped only four times the seed that they sowed. In later centuries, especially from the second century AD onward, conditions became still worse. Many farms were utterly abandoned; the land was concentrated in the hands of a comparatively few large proprietors. The tenants fell into chronic debt and were little better than slaves. So eager were many of them to escape from the thralldom in which their poverty kept them that they flocked to the cities, until laws were passed which bound them to the soil as serfs. All these and many other evil consequences appear to have flowed from a widespread decline in agriculture, which, though alleviated at times, grew worse and worse until Rome finally fell.

The difference between Roman agriculture in early and in later times has given rise to a warm debate. One side is represented by Durneau de la Malle. As he put it: "A vicious system of agriculture, a biennial rotation, the ignorance of the methods of alternation of crops, the too frequent rotation of wheat on the same land, the insufficient and poor preparation of manure, the slight extent of artificial grasslands, the small number of animals supported on cultivated crops, the imperfection of the methods and instruments of culture, the vicious practice of burning the straw in place of converting it into manure, these and a hundred other deadly practices which it would be too long to enumerate form the conflicting but true picture which Greek and Roman agriculture on the whole present to us." Rodbertus strongly contested this view. He attempted to show that the Romans had a most admirable system of agriculture, being familiar with the rotation of crops and the use of fertilizers, and that more labor was expended per acre than is now spent on the best fields of Germany. That there was agricultural decline he admitted, but he ascribed it to social causes. In the writings of such men as Varro, Cato, Pliny, and Columella, he accepts the parts which indicate that the science of agriculture was highly developed, but says that other portions must be taken "cum grano sallis." He thinks the Latin writers have been misunderstood or that their statements can be explained by other circumstances. For instance, he supposes that when Rome was able to reach out and obtain grain from other lands the Italian farmers turned their attention to vineyards, olive orchards, and cattle raising, and only the worst fields in Italy were devoted to wheat. Hence it was not surprising that the farmers reaped only four times what they had sowed.

Professor Simkhovitch ably shows that these two views are not really contradictory. The picture painted by Rodbertus indicates the condition in the early days, when Rome was in her prime. The other presents the conditions of later times. Simkhovitch ascribes the difference to exhaustion of the soil. Such exhaustion, as he says, is not a necessary consequence of incorrect cultivation, but arises only when unwise methods are pursued. As Van Hise I points out, the most crucial element in the exhaustion of the soil is the depletion of the phosphorus, which can be prevented only by abundant fertilization.

171. Which answer accurately describes the nature of the evidence used in the text?
    a. Studies of the physical earth that date back to the time of ancient civilizations
    b. Multiple papers published on the idea of climate change and agricultural exhaustion
    c. Textual evidence, observations, and historical records of Roman observers
    d. Accounts of Rome's decline from enemy sources

172. Based on the information in the passage, which answer could best quantify the effect agricultural decline had on the fall of Rome?

    a. The lack of good land to harvest grain contributed to the food shortages that taxed Rome's resources to the brink and brought about economic and civil degradation.

    b. Rome became dependent on other lands for grain, making the empire less reliant on its own resources and prone to collapse.

    c. The Roman empire collapsed as it struggled to maintain economic prosperity.

    d. Lacking sufficient means to feed its armies, Rome could not withstand the attacks of barbarian tribes.

173. Which information serves as the best evidence supporting Rodbertus' following claim about agricultural decline?

    "Rodbertus strongly contested this view. He attempted to show that the Romans had a most admirable system of agriculture, being familiar with the rotation of crops and the use of fertilizers, and that more labor was expended per acre than is now spent on the best fields of Germany. That there was agricultural decline he admitted, but he ascribed it to social causes."

    a. A series of severe droughts was reported within Rome's last fifteen years of power.

    b. Rome sought to colonize other areas of the empire, so many Roman farmers moved to the frontiers.

    c. Evidence was found that Romans developed agricultural systems that harvested steady grain supplies even in low yields.

    d. Increasing land taxes led to farmers having dwindling resources to produce crops and overworking the land.

174. Huntignton brings in the perspectives of several scholars. Some of his sources support his views, and some disagree with the idea of agricultural decline resulting in the fall of Rome. What does this do for the author's argument?

    a. This weakens the argument and confuses the reader; clearly, there are scholars who provide reasons that agricultural decline was not the cause of the fall of the Roman empire.

    b. This allows the author to provide a full scope of the idea to the audience; by addressing the conflicting views, he can strengthen his ideas by showing how logic or other evidence shows gaps within the insight of the opposing views.

    c. This does nothing for the argument; the author has no argument but to elaborate on a specific historical theory.

    d. The author is showing how unfounded the opposing views to the agricultural decline theory are.

175. What can be inferred from the following excerpt?

    "Professor Simkhovitch ably shows that these two views are not really contradictory. The picture painted by Rodbertus indicates the condition in the early days, when Rome was in her prime. The other presents the conditions of later times. Simkhovitch ascribes the difference to exhaustion of the soil. Such exhaustion, as he says, is not a necessary consequence of wrong cultivation, but arises only when unwise methods are pursued."

    a. Periods of agricultural decline were not uncommon in ancient Rome.

    b. Rodbertus' view focuses on an earlier irrelevant time in Rome's history.

    c. Romans were actually unskilled at farming.

    d. Soil exhaustion can occur instantaneously from unwise methods.

176. What's the best way for the author to consolidate the following details into an argument for agricultural decline leading to Rome's collapse?

"In later centuries, especially from the second century AD onward, conditions became still worse. Many farms were utterly abandoned; the land was concentrated in the hands of a comparatively few large proprietors. The tenants fell into chronic debt and were little better than slaves. So eager were many of them to escape from the thralldom in which their poverty kept them that they flocked to the cities, until laws were passed which bound them to the soil as serfs."

a. Because the farmers were so poor, they could not adequately produce crops needed to sustain the empire.
b. The fact that farmers were abandoning their land suggests increasing soil infertility; the Romans became dependent on other sources of food.
c. The evidence suggests that soil conditions were consistently declining to the point that the government had to enforce laws to try and keep people working the land to try and grow food.
d. The first century AD was Rome's greatest crop yield.

The following passage is an excerpt from "The Christian Coloring in the Beowulf," by F. A. Blackburn. Pleaes read it and answer questions 177 – 182.

It is admitted by all critics that the Beowulf is essentially a heathen poem; that its materials are drawn from tales composed before the conversion of the Angles and Saxons to Christianity, and that there was a time when these tales were repeated without the Christian reflections and allusions that are found in the poem that has reached us. But in what form this heathen material existed before it was put into its present shape is a question on which opinions are widely different. In the nature of the case we can look for no entire consensus of opinion and no exact answer to the question; the most that one can expect to establish is at the best only a probability.

The following hypotheses are possible: 1. The poem was composed by a Christian, who had heard the stories and used them as the material for his work. 2. The poem was composed by a Christian, who used old lays as his material. (This differs from the first supposition in assuming that the tales had already been versified and were in poetical form before they were used by the author.) 3. The poem was composed by a heathen, either from old stories or from old lays. At a later date, it was revised by a Christian poet, to whom we owe the Christian allusions found in it. (This hypothesis differs from the others in assuming the existence of a complete poem without the Christian coloring.)

The purpose of the present study is to contribute to the settlement of the question inferences drawn from a careful examination of the passages that show a Christian coloring. Whether the Beowulf is a unit or a compilation made from several poems originally distinct is not considered, except in so far as a conclusion may be drawn from the character of the Christian allusions, and all other questions in regard to the genesis of the Epic in general or of the Beowulf in particular are also left untouched.

It must be noted, however, at the beginning of the discussion, that it is not in all cases a simple matter to decide whether a passage under consideration is Christian in character. It is clear, I think, that we have no right to classify under this head those passages that are simply moral and ethical. The commandment not to bear false witness is regarded with good reason as a fundamental part of Christian doctrine, but when the dying Beowulf says, "I sought not unrighteous strife nor swore oaths deceitfully," we are justified in claiming the passage as Christian only by bringing proof that our fore- fathers, before they were enlightened by the instruction of Christian missionaries, thought false oaths right and proper. But when the hero continues, "In all this I may rejoice, though sick with mortal wounds, for when my life hath left my body, the Ruler of men may not charge me with the murder of my kindred," we may properly recognize the Christian coloring. This does not lie in the assertion of the speaker that he has kept the commandment not to kill, for Christianity can claim a monopoly of this no more than of the other just referred to, but in the apparent reference to a judgment after death and to the Ruler who is to try men for their deeds; a reference that seems to prove the writer's knowledge of the teaching of the Gospels.

Other passages are doubtful for a different reason. It is well known that the missionaries of the early Church took many words belonging to heathen beliefs and practices and applied them to corresponding conceptions and usages of the Christian system. In Yule, Easter, God, hell, etc., we still keep words thus adopted; others, now obsolete, are hcelend, nergend, drihten, metod, frea, etc. To these may be added the various epithets applied to the Persons of the Trinity, which are used so freely by the Old English poets. Most of these are simply equivalents of Latin expressions, or imitations of them; e.g., celmihtig (omnipotens); ece drihten (dominus seternus); wuldorcyning (rex glorise); and the like. This use of native words and epithets is nothing peculiar, of course; the same thing had already taken place in Latin and had given to deus, dominus, etc., their ecclesiastical meaning. But when such words are first used by the church, it is plain that something of the old meaning still clings to them and is suggested to the hearer. In some cases, the older meaning vanishes after a time or becomes entirely subordinated to the later one; e.g., the word Christ has entirely lost, for most of those that use or hear it, its original meaning; God and Saviour have the older and more general meaning at times, but more often the later specialized one; Father and Son, as names of the Persons of the Trinity, are far less frequent than as ordinary names of relationship. We cannot always feel certain, therefore, in reading the Beowulf, whether the word is used by the writer with full consciousness of its later sense or with its older meaning. All cases of this kind are included in the following discussion; the question whether the earlier or the later meaning is to be assumed is considered in its place. There are in the Beowulf sixty-eight passages in which the form of expression or the character of the thought seems to suggest something in Christian usage or doctrine, and we may properly assume that they had this effect on Christian readers at the time that the manuscript that has reached us was written. These passages may be classified according to content as follows: 1. Passages containing Bible history or allusions to some Scripture narrative. 2. Passages containing expressions in disapproval of heathen ideas or heathen worship. 3. Passages containing references to doctrines distinctively Christian. 4. Incidental allusions to the Christian God, to his attributes, and to his part in shaping the lives and fortunes of men. The fourth class is by far the most numerous; it comprises fifty-three cases . . .

177. What is the author's primary stance on the origins of *Beowulf*?
   a. The writer believes that the writer of *Beowulf* was a Christian who compiled old lays of pagan poetry and inserted Christian references in key areas.
   b. The author was probably a pagan convert to Christianity.
   c. The text was adapted from a finished pagan text.
   d. The author doesn't state his personal stance but rather explores the different possibilities of *Beowulf*'s origins.

178. Why might the author have thought the use of "coloring" for his title was an appropriate word choice?

    a. *Beowulf* is a story; this would enable the work to identify with the interest of children who may want to read the text.

    b. This is a nod to the Christian elements and themes that were inserted into the original pagan text.

    c. This reflects how the pagan concepts in the text were completely covered up by Christian symbolism.

    d. This is a metaphor for the way the story of Beowulf colors vivid imagery in the reader's mind.

179. What inference can be made on the nature of morality presented in the following text?

    "It is clear, I think, that we have no right to classify under this head those passages that are simply moral and ethical. The commandment not to bear false witness is regarded with good reason as a fundamental part of Christian doctrine, but when the dying Beowulf says, 'I sought not unrighteous strife nor swore oaths deceitfully,' we are justified in claiming the passage as Christian only by bringing proof that our fore-fathers, before they were enlightened by the instruction of Christian missionaries, thought false oaths right and proper."

    a. There are common moral principles in pagan and Christian cultures.

    b. Christian excerpts are only present when citing the Ten Commandments in specific terms.

    c. Pagans had identical moral values.

    d. Christians brought morality to the pagans.

180. Which revelation would prove beyond a doubt that the following second theory was the actual origin of *Beowulf*'s development?

    "The poem was composed by a Christian, who used old lays as his material" (the tales had already been versified and were in poetical form before they were used by the author).

    a. A medieval etching depicting a scribe writing the epic on vellum

    b. Medieval chronicles documenting an instance of a pagan storyteller visiting the monastery where *Beowulf* was written down

    c. Documents discovered that chronicle a monk's effort to organize Anglo-Saxon poems based on Beowulf myths

    d. An account written by a monk that recalls a story from one of the recent converts about an ancient hero named Beowulf

181. Which *best* explains the reasoning/motivation behind the writer of *Beowulf* using "passages containing expressions in disapproval of heathen ideas or heathen worship"?

    a. To assert that heathen ideals are sinful

    b. To discredit pagan ideas and perspectives and elevate Christian virtues and worship

    c. To assert the power of the church

    d. To create a story that highlights Christian ideals

182. The concept of wyrd, or fate, remains as a recurring pagan theme within *Beowulf*. Which explanation might the author use to address the presence of fate in *Beowulf*?

a. Fate is a concept shared by Christians and pagans, so the author left the references to fate.

b. A mistranslation is probably why "fate" remains in the text.

c. Fate brings in mind damnation or the cost of living in sin; therefore, the author left it as a way to keep readers focused on following Christian doctrine.

d. The author might not have fully understood the concept of pagan fate but worked it into the text in a way that it could be seen as divine providence or God's will.

The following passage is an excerpt from "The Pose of Sauropodous Dinosaurs," by Dr. W.D. Matthew. Please read it and answer questions 183 – 188.

These four articles discuss a question of considerable general interest. Did the huge Sauropodous dinosaurs, Diplodocus, Brontosaurus, and their allies, walk like elephants, or crawl like crocodiles? The skeletons and casts in the larger museums of America and Europe have all been mounted straight limbed, with the body well clear of the ground. But the evidence for giving them this pose, so different from that of the generality of reptiles, although well known to those who are responsible for it, has not, until recently, been published. Hence it is not surprising that these reconstructions have been criticized more or less seriously, especially in Germany, and that two writers of high scientific standing—Dr. Tornier in Berlin, and Dr. Hay in Washington—have contended that these animals could not have walked upright, but must have dragged the belly on the ground as crocodiles and lizards normally do. Both writers have attempted and discussed at length the re-articulation of the skeleton in the crocodilian pose.

Dr. Tornier's argument is, briefly, that reptiles crawl while mammals walk; that Diplodocus is a reptile and resembles the lizards and crocodiles far more closely than it does any mammals in the details of construction of the shoulder and hip-girdles, limbs, and feet. Therefore, it should be posed like one of the larger lizards, except for the long neck, which he compares to the long-necked birds and poses in accordance. A sketch restoration and a number of diagrammatic drawings illustrate his views. The subject appears, frankly, to be somewhat outside the range of his studies, and his comparisons are not broad or thorough enough to be at all convincing.

His criticisms are very effectively and completely answered by Dr. Abel and Dr. Holland. These authors point out that while the dinosaurs were reptiles and as such their bones were constructed upon the reptilian plan, yet they form a group apart, differing from other reptiles and in many respects resembling the struthious birds; that these resemblances, especially as regards the construction of pelvis and hind limbs, leave no reasonable doubt that the typical dinosaurs walked pretty much as do the great ground birds; that the limbs of Diplodocus and its allies differ from the normal dinosaur type in a marked superficial and adaptive resemblance to the elephant, indicating a quadrupedal "rectigrade" mode of motion; that the skeleton articulates satisfactorily in this pose and that the attempt to articulate it in the pose of a crocodile or lizard involves either a demonstrably false interpretation of parts, or a disarticulation of the joints which proves such a position to be highly abnormal if not utterly impossible for the creature to assume.

Dr. Hay's contributions to the discussion—the article cited and an earlier one in the American Naturalist—are worthy of more careful consideration. Hay is a high authority on fossil vertebrate, especially upon Chelonia and fishes, and has recently devoted considerable study to the dinosaurs. He recognizes the fact that the dinosaurs, while pertaining to the class Reptilia, form a group apart, with many analogies to the birds; that many dinosaurs did walk with the body clear of the ground, and that many lizards walk or run in this way at times. He does not deny that even the Sauropocla may have done so at times, but regards them as too massive and heavy for this to have been their normal mode of progress. But his chief protest is against the placing of the knee and elbow joints in sagittal planes (i.e., bending parallel with the middle line of the body) as in mammals, instead of bending outward as in all modern reptiles. In certain points of his argument he makes out a convincing case in the reviewer's opinion; other points may be satisfactorily answered.

Dr. Hay misstates the supposed significance of the peculiar type of femur seen in Diplodocus. He observes:

> If the mammal-like gait of Diplodocus be insisted upon the ground of straightness of the femur, it may be pointed out . . . that the femora of Sphenodon and of lizards, animals that creep, are straight. If it be contended that it is in the heavy-bodied animals that a straight femur is correlated with a lifting of the body from the ground during locomotion, it may be permitted to recall that the femora of Allosaurus and Tyrannosaurus, great carnivorous dinosaurs, are distinctly bent. The femora of Trachodon are straight, while those of Camptosaurus and Laosaurnts are curved. Curvature of the femur seems therefore to have no relation to size of body or erectness of pose.

But no one, so far as the reviewer knows, has asserted that the straightness of the shaft of the femur of Diplodocus, considered alone, provide that the animal walked like a mammal. For among mammals there are both straight and curved femora, and a wide variety of gaits.

183. What seems to be the root of the debate between how *Sauropodous* dinosaurs stood and moved?
    a. Scientists of the time identified dinosaurs as reptiles, but there is evidence to suggest that they weren't structured like modern reptiles, fueling contention on the subject.
    b. Dinosaurs seem to have birdlike qualities and reptilian qualities, so scientists argue about whether dinosaurs were more like birds or reptiles.
    c. The bone structures are so unique that it's hard to tell.
    d. There is no way to properly gauge how the animals moved.

184. Based on the information in the third paragraph, which mostly likely describes the word *rectigrade*?
    a. Rectangular
    b. Straight
    c. Sideways
    d. Circular

185. Which statement would the author most likely agree with?
    a. Dinosaurs might be warm-blooded.
    b. Dinosaurs are not reptiles at all.
    c. Large animals share physical structures and movement patterns.
    d. Dinosaurs have commonalities with modern reptiles, but they clearly belong to a different category.

186. The author has decided to add details on fossilized *Diplodocus* footprints as potential evidence of how they moved. Where would this information best fit in the piece?

a. Opening with footprint evidence would present the debate between dinosaur movements more clearly.

b. This information would be very good toward the end of this passage, introducing new evidence aside from bones.

c. These details should be added after the third paragraph.

d. This information should be inserted after the second paragraph.

187. What can be inferred from the following statement?

"But no one, so far as the reviewer knows, has asserted that the straightness of the shaft of the femur of Diplodocus, considered alone, provide that the animal walked like a mammal. For among mammals there are both straight and curved femora, and a wide variety of gaits."

a. *Diplodocus* could have had curved femur.

b. *Diplodocus* could have had a range of movements.

c. The shape of the femur doesn't solely define body movement.

d. Most dinosaurs probably moved more like mammals.

188. The writer presents the views of multiple scientists in the passage. Does he seem to side with one particular scientist more than any other?

a. The writer is completely unbiased with no favoritism.

b. He clearly favors Dr. Tornier's argument.

c. He sides more with Dr. Hay.

d. The author seems to think Dr. Abel and Dr. Holland have a stronger case.

The following passage is an excerpt from "Natural Law," by Oliver Wendell Holmes. Please read it and answer questions 189 – 194.

The jurists who believe in natural law seem to me to be in that naive state of mind that accepts what has been familiar and accepted by them and their neighbors as something that must be accepted by all men everywhere. No doubt it is true that, so far as we can see ahead, some arrangements and the rudiments of familiar institutions seem to be necessary elements in any society that may spring from our own and that would seem to us to be civilized—some form of permanent association between the sexes—some residue of property individually owned—some mode of binding oneself to specified future conduct—at the bottom of all, some protection for the person. But without speculating whether a group is imaginable in which all but the last of these might disappear and the last be subject to qualifications that most of us would abhor, the question remains as to the Ought of natural law.

It is true that beliefs and wishes have a transcendental basis in the sense that their foundation is arbitrary. You cannot help entertaining and feeling them, and there is an end of it. As an arbitrary fact people wish to live, and we say with various degrees of certainty that they can do so only on certain conditions. To do it they must eat and drink. That necessity is absolute. It is a necessity of less degree but practically general that they should live in society. If they live in society, so far as we can see, there are further conditions. Reason working on experience does tell us, no doubt, that if our wish to live continues, we can do it only on those terms. But that seems to me the whole of the matter. I see no a priori duty to live with others and in that way, but simply a statement of what I must do if I wish to remain alive. If I do live with others they tell me that I must do and abstain from doing various things or they will put the screws on to me. I believe that they will, and being of the same mind as to their conduct I not only accept the rules but come in time to accept them with sympathy and emotional affirmation and begin to talk about duties and rights. But for legal purposes a right is only the hypostasis of a prophecy—the imagination of a substance supporting the fact that the public force will be brought to bear upon those who do things said to contravene it—just as we talk of the force of gravitation accounting for the conduct of bodies in space. One phrase adds no more than the other to what we know without it. No doubt behind these legal rights is the fighting will of the subject to maintain them, and the spread of his emotions to the general rules by which they are maintained; but that does not seem to me the same thing as the supposed a priori discernment of a duty or the assertion of a preexisting right. A dog will fight for his bone.

The most fundamental of the supposed pre-existing rights—the right to life—is sacrificed without a scruple not only in war, but whenever the interest of society, that is, of the predominant power in the community, is thought to demand it. Whether that interest is the interest of mankind in the long run no one can tell, and as, in any event, to those who do not think with Kant and Hegel it is only an interest, the sanctity disappears. I remember a very tender-hearted judge being of opinion that closing a hatch to stop a fire and the destruction of a cargo was justified even if it was known that doing so would stifle a man below. It is idle to illustrate further, because to those who agree with me I am uttering commonplaces and to those who disagree I am ignoring the necessary foundations of thought. The a priori men generally call the dissentients superficial. But I do agree with them in believing that one's attitude on these matters is closely connected with one's general attitude toward the universe. Proximately, as has been suggested, it is determined largely by early associations and temperament, coupled with the desire to have an absolute guide. Men to a great extent believe what they want to—although I see in that no basis for a philosophy that tells us what we should want to want.

189. What is the author's point of the following sentence?
     "It is true that beliefs and wishes have a transcendental basis in the sense that their foundation is arbitrary."

a. Beliefs and wishes are not real.
b. Beliefs are naturally arbitrary; this shouldn't be used to create laws.
c. Beliefs and wishes are only true in the sense that humans believe in them and give them validation based on personal views.
d. Wishes can become beliefs, which then become real, when people enact laws and circumstances to make them so.

190. What seems to be the core concept of the author's argument?
a. Laws are subjective constructions made by humans, so there's no force binding these things to reality.
b. There is no free will.
c. Natural law is good but not universal.
d. Universal law is inherently oppressive because some people are against natural law.

191. What would be the best way to counter the author's argument?
    a. Examples of shared values and beliefs are evident around the world.
    b. Nature seems bound by certain principles, so one can infer that civilization functions around a core of natural laws binding it together.
    c. His argument is rendered moot because it's essentially an opinion based on his own experience; it can't be used to judge the views or beliefs of others.
    d. Immanuel Kant's "I think therefore I am"; if people believe and want natural laws to be present and live by them, they can act in a way that reality conforms to this idea. People can make natural law true.

192. What might be a flaw in the author's use of the following example as evidence to support his belief that the "right to life" concept within natural law has no hold in reality?
    "I remember a very tender-hearted judge being of opinion that closing a hatch to stop a fire and the destruction of a cargo was justified even if it was known that doing so would stifle a man below."

    a. Judges are bound to uphold natural law; this example is still just.
    b. Natural law upholds the common good; this is a case on a smaller scale than the overall good of humanity.
    c. The men might not have died, which wouldn't make this murder.
    d. The author does not consider the reasoning behind the judge or the people involved.

193. Based on this article, what can we infer about the author?
    a. He probably believes that laws are ultimately useless.
    b. He probably believes upbringing, not inherent nature, molds the individual.
    c. He is probably a defense lawyer.
    d. He probably believes human cognition is what defines us as a species.

194. In the following passage, how does the author believe laws work?
    "But for legal purposes a right is only the hypostasis of a prophecy—the imagination of a substance supporting the fact that the public force will be brought to bear upon those who do things said to contravene it."

    a. Laws are fictional; they have no basis in reality.
    b. Laws are based on fear of repercussion.
    c. Laws can be manipulated according to insights or beliefs.
    d. Laws exist only because humans create them and are followed out of fear of going against the mass supporting the laws.

The following passage is an excerpt from "The Theme of Paradise Lost," by H. W. Peck. Please read it and answer questions 195 –200.

The most widely accepted, and what was for a long time the orthodox theory, is that Paradise Lost is a theological and historical epic, dealing with human and super-human facts, its action beginning before the creation, and ending with the disposition of things for eternity. Its central conceptions are the truths of Christianity, represented with splendor of language, and in certain portions with wealth of poetic ornament. The attitude of earlier critics who accepted this view was, in the main, one of unstinted admiration. Dennis and Addison may be taken as representatives. Even Dr. Johnson, who was bitterly opposed to Milton on the subject of politics,

118

and out of sympathy with many of the traits of his character, yet reverenced his achievement in Paradise Lost, and mentioned as an undisputed fact that the substance of the narrative is truth.

But with the nineteenth century there came a different view of the universe. Biblical criticism and the advance of scientific knowledge made it impossible for many to accept as literal truth the Biblical account of the creation and the fall. The matter of Paradise Lost is consequently to be discarded, and the fame of the poem is to rest upon the sublimity and harmony of its style. The chief representative of this class of critics is Edmond Scherer.

Another variety of the critical opinion which considers that in substance Paradise Lost is theological and historical is found in Mark Pattison's work on Milton: "Milton's mental constitution, then, demanded in the material upon which it was to work, a combination of qualities such as very few subjects could offer. The events and person—ages must be real and substantial, for he could not occupy himself seriously with airy nothings and creatures of pure fancy. Yet they must not be such events and personages as history had portrayed to us with well-known characters, and all their virtues, faults, foibles, and peculiarities. And, lastly, it was requisite that they should be the common property and the familiar interest of a wide circle of English readers."

Again: "The world of Paradise Lost is an ideal, conventional world, quite as much as the world of the Arabian Nights, or the world of the chivalrous romance, or that of the pastoral novel. Not only dramatic, but all, poetry is founded on illusion. We must, though it be but for the moment, suppose it true. We must be transported out of the actual world into that world in which the given scene is laid." The inconsistency in these passages is significant; the writer seems to be following two divergent paths, historical accuracy, and purely literary appreciation.

A second class of critics, who believe that the Biblical account of the creation and the fall is a myth, yet who have been deeply impressed by the grandeur of Milton's epic, have resorted to another method of interpretation. Assuming that Milton's avowed purpose to "assert Eternal Providence, and justify the ways of God to men" was a misconception of the true spirit of his undertaking, they consider the epic to be chiefly symbolic and poetic. On this view, the poet himself may not be fully conscious of his own deeper meaning. Among this class are those who hold that the subject of the poem is the revolt of Lucifer; that Satan is the hero; and the central idea, the struggle of liberty against authority.

The romantic poets of the nineteenth century, especially Byron and Shelley, accepted this interpretation; and it is congenial to the more recent idealization of the Superman. Readers of Jack London will recall in The Sea-Wolf the admiration of Wolf Larsen for those passages in which Satan is the dominating figure.

A contemporary essayist holds that the "true theme is Paradise itself "; that the profound value and interest of the epic resides in its poetic realization of the ideal of pastoral literature in the portrayal of the Eden bower.

195. Which phrase best describes the author's main objective in the passage?
    a. He seeks to identify the true theme of *Paradise Lost*.
    b. He seeks to explain the theme of *Paradise Lost* to the readers who might not know about it.
    c. He seeks to explore the various interpretations of *Paradise Lost*'s theme in an effort to consolidate the work's primary meaning.
    d. He seeks to prove that *Paradise Lost* can only be understood when the reader acknowledges that for Milton the content is historically accurate and real.

196. The author incorporates the views of several writers from different eras to discuss *Paradise Lost*'s themes. Why might the author choose to use this in his work?
    a. This highlights how much Milton's masterpiece has remained relevant.
    b. This serves both to show the wide range of artistic interpretations of Milton, as well as how the text has been received throughout time.
    c. Many writers have been influenced by Milton; several of them have had altering views on the theme of the text, which appear in their works.
    d. The fact that many writers have views on Milton highlights the wide debate over the theme of the text.

197. Which of the following terms could best replace "mental constitution" used in the third paragraph?
    a. Interests
    b. Sanity
    c. State of mind
    d. Brain composition

198. If Milton had written passages with unconscious symbolism, as mentioned in the sixth paragraph, what could be inferred about *Paradise Lost*?
    a. Milton is a clear master of symbolism.
    b. This symbolism present in the work must be discarded; only literal interpretations prevail.
    c. *Paradise Lost*'s theme in itself may be inconsequential.
    d. If people can interpret symbolism when Milton might not have intended, the theme itself is subjective to a degree.

199. Truth seems to be a major focus of this essay fragment. Based on what the author writes, is it conceivable that *Paradise Lost* may contain multiple layers of truth?
    a. No. It's clear that *Paradise Lost*'s core truth is that it's intended to assert "eternal Providence, and justify the ways of God to men."
    b. Yes. Milton clearly was a master of poetry and the use of symbolic metaphors and allusions.
    c. Yes. Conceivably, Milton intended a literal truth in his work while intentionally commenting and focusing on other themes in addition to theology.
    d. No. It's very likely that Milton wanted to address the single truth: the fall of man chronicled in the Bible.

200. The author has decided to incorporate a section on how Milton's epic style lends itself to the interpretation of the text and key characters. Where would this information best serve the text?
    a. Just after the fifth paragraph
    b. At the beginning of the passage
    c. At the conclusion of the passage
    d. Between the sixth and seventh paragraphs

Answer Explanations

1. C: The author contrasts two different viewpoints, then builds a case showing preference for one over the other. Choice *A* is incorrect because the introduction does not contain an impartial definition, but rather, an opinion. Choice *B* is incorrect. There is no puzzling phenomenon given, as the author doesn't mention any peculiar cause or effect that is in question regarding poetry. Choice *D* does contain another's viewpoint at the beginning of the passage; however, to say that the author has no stake in this argument is incorrect; the author uses personal experiences to build their case.

2. B: Choice *B* accurately describes the author's argument in the text: that poetry is not irrelevant. While the author does praise, and even value, Buddy Wakefield as a poet, the author never heralds him as a genius. Eliminate Choice *A*, as it is an exaggeration. Not only is Choice *C* an exaggerated statement, but the author never mentions spoken word poetry in the text. Choice *D* is wrong because this statement contradicts the writer's argument.

3. D: *Exiguously* means not occurring often, or occurring rarely, so Choice *D* would LEAST change the meaning of the sentence. Choice *A*, *indolently*, means unhurriedly, or slow, and does not fit the context of the sentence. Choice *B*, *inaudibly*, means quietly or silently. Choice *C*, *interminably*, means endlessly, or all the time, and is the opposite of the word *exiguously*.

4. D: A student's insistence that psychoanalysis is a subset of modern psychology is the most analogous option. The author of the passage tries to insist that performance poetry is a subset of modern poetry, and therefore, tries to prove that modern poetry is not "dying," but thriving on social media for the masses. Choice *A* is incorrect, as the author is not refusing any kind of validation. Choice *B* is incorrect; the author's insistence is that poetry will *not* lose popularity. Choice *C* mimics the topic but compares two different genres, while the author does no comparison in this passage.

5. B: The author's purpose is to disprove Gioia's article claiming that poetry is a dying art form that only survives in academic settings. In order to prove his argument, the author educates the reader about new developments in poetry (Choice *A*) and describes the brilliance of a specific modern poet (Choice *C*), but these serve as examples of a growing poetry trend that counters Gioia's argument. Choice *D* is incorrect because it contradicts the author's argument.

6. D: This question is difficult because the choices offer real reasons as to why the author includes the quote. However, the question specifically asks for the *main reason* for including the quote. The quote from a recently written poem shows that people are indeed writing, publishing, and performing poetry (Choice *B*). The quote also shows that people are still listening to poetry (Choice *C*). These things are true, and by their nature, serve to disprove Gioia's views (Choice *A*), which is the author's goal. However, Choice *D* is the most direct reason for including the quote, because the article analyzes the quote for its "complex themes" that "draws listeners and appreciation" right after it's given.

7. C: *Extraneous* most nearly means *superfluous*, or *trivial*. Choice *A*, *indispensable*, is incorrect because it means the opposite of *extraneous*. Choice *B, bewildering*, means *confusing* and is not relevant to the context of the sentence. Finally, Choice *D* is wrong because although the prefix of the word is the same, *ex-*, the word *exuberant* means *elated* or *enthusiastic*, and is irrelevant to the context of the sentence.

8. A: The author's purpose is to bring to light an alternative view on human perception by examining the role of technology in human understanding. This is a challenging question because the author's purpose is somewhat open-ended. The author concludes by stating that the questions regarding human perception and observation can be approached from many angles. Thus, the author does not seem to be attempting to prove one thing or another. Choice *B* is clearly wrong because we cannot know for certain whether the electron experiment is the latest discovery in astroparticle physics because no date is given. Choice *C* is a broad generalization that does not reflect accurately on the writer's views. While the author does appear to reflect on opposing views of human understanding (Choice *D*), the best answer is Choice *A*.

9. C: It presents a problem, explains the details of that problem, and then ends with more inquiry. The beginning of this paragraph literally "presents a conundrum," explains the problem of partial understanding, and then ends with more questions, or inquiry. There is no solution offered in this paragraph, making Choices *A and B* incorrect. Choice *D* is incorrect because the paragraph does not begin with a definition.

10. D: Looking back in the text, the author describes that classical philosophy holds that understanding can be reached by careful observation. This will not work if they are overly invested or biased in their pursuit. Choices *A*, *B*, and *C* are in no way related and are completely unnecessary. A specific theory is not necessary to understanding, according to classical philosophy mentioned by the author.

11. B: The electrons passed through both holes and then onto the plate. Choices *A* and *C* are wrong because such movement is not mentioned at all in the text. In the passage the author says that electrons that were physically observed appeared to pass through one hole or another. Remember, the electrons that were observed doing this were described as acting like particles. Therefore, Choice *D* is wrong. Recall that the plate actually recorded electrons passing through both holes simultaneously and hitting the plate. This behavior, the electron activity that wasn't seen by humans, was characteristic of waves. Thus, Choice *B* is the right answer.

12. C: The author mentions "gravity" to demonstrate an example of natural phenomena humans discovered and understand without the use of tools or machines. Choice *A* mirrors the language in the beginning of the paragraph, but is incorrect in its intent. Choice *B* is incorrect; the paragraph mentions nothing of "not knowing the true nature of gravity." Choice *D* and *E* is incorrect as well. There is no mention of an "alternative solution" in this paragraph.

13. A: The important thing to keep in mind is that we must choose a scenario that best parallels, or is most similar to, the discovery of the experiment mentioned in the passage. The important aspects of the experiment can be summed up like so: humans directly observed one behavior of electrons and then through analyzing a tool (the plate that recorded electron hits), discovered that there was another electron behavior that could not be physically seen by human eyes. This summary best parallels the scenario in Choice *A*. Like Feynman, the colorblind person can observe one aspect of the world but through the special goggles (a tool), he is able to see a natural phenomenon that he could not physically see on his own. While Choice *D* is compelling, the x-ray helps humans see the broken bone, but it does not necessarily reveal that the bone is broken in the first place. The other choices do not parallel the scenario in question. Therefore, Choice *A* is the best choice.

14. B: The author would not agree that technology renders human observation irrelevant. Choice *A* is incorrect because much of the passage discusses how technology helps humans observe what cannot be seen with the naked eye; therefore, the author would agree with this statement. This line of reasoning is also why the author would agree with Choice *D*, making it incorrect as well. As indicated in the second paragraph, the author seems to think that humans create inventions and tools with the goal of studying phenomena more precisely. This indicates increased understanding as people recognize limitations and develop items to help bypass the limitations and learn. Therefore, Choice C is incorrect as well. Again, the author doesn't attempt to disprove or dismiss classical philosophy.

15. D: The author explains that Boethianism is a Medieval theological philosophy that attributes sin to temporary pleasure and righteousness with virtue and God's providence. Besides Choice D, the choices listed are all physical things. While these could still be divine rewards, Boethianism holds that the true reward for being virtuous is in God's favor. It is also stressed in the article that physical pleasures cannot be taken into the afterlife. Therefore, the best choice is D, God's favor.

16. C: *The Canterbury Tales* presents a manuscript written in the medieval period that can help illustrate Boethianism through stories and show how people of the time might have responded to the idea. Choices A and B are generalized statements, and we have no evidence to support Choice B. Choice D is very compelling, but it looks at Boethianism in a way that the author does not. The author does not mention "different levels of Boethianism" when discussing the tales, only that the concept appears differently in different tales. Boethianism also doesn't focus on enlightenment.

17. D: The author is referring to the principle that a desire for material goods leads to moral malfeasance punishable by a higher being. Choice A is incorrect; while the text does mention thieves ravaging others' possessions, it is only meant as an example and not as the principle itself. Choice B is incorrect for the same reason as A. Choice C is mentioned in the text and is part of the example that proves the principle, and also not the principle itself.

18. C: The word *avarice* most nearly means *parsimoniousness*, or an unwillingness to spend money. Choice A means *evil* or *mischief* and does not relate to the context of the sentence. Choice B is also incorrect, because *pithiness* means *shortness* or *conciseness*. Choice D is close because *precariousness* means dangerous or instability, which goes well with the context. However, we are told of the summoner's specific characteristic of greed, which makes Choice C the best answer.

19. D: Desire for pleasure can lead toward sin. Boethianism acknowledges desire as something that leads out of holiness, so Choice A is incorrect. Choice B is incorrect because in the passage, Boethianism is depicted as being wary of desire and anything that binds people to the physical world. Choice C can be eliminated because the author never says that desire indicates demonic.

20. A: The purpose is to inform the reader about what assault is and how it is committed. Choice B is incorrect because the passage does not state that assault is a lesser form of lethal force, only that an assault can use lethal force, or alternatively, lethal force can be utilized to counter a dangerous assault. Choice C is incorrect because the passage is informative and does not have a set agenda. Finally, Choice D is incorrect because although the author uses an example in order to explain assault, it is not indicated that this is the author's personal account.

21. C: If the man being attacked in an alley by another man with a knife used self-defense by lethal force, it would not be considered illegal. The presence of a deadly weapon indicates mal-intent and because the individual is isolated in an alley, lethal force in self-defense may be the only way to preserve his life. Choices A and B can be ruled out because in these situations, no one is in danger of immediate death or bodily harm by someone else. Choice D is an assault and does exhibit intent to harm, but this situation isn't severe enough to merit lethal force; there is no intent to kill.

22. B: As discussed in the second passage, there are several forms of assault, like assault with a deadly weapon, verbal assault, or threatening posture or language. Choice A is incorrect because the author does mention what the charges are on assaults; therefore, we cannot assume that they are more or less

123

than unnecessary use of force charges. Choice *C* is incorrect because anyone is capable of assault; the author does not state that one group of people cannot commit assault. Choice *D* is incorrect because assault is never justified. Self-defense resulting in lethal force can be justified.

23. D: The use of lethal force is not evaluated on the intent of the user, but rather on the severity of the primary attack that warranted self-defense. This statement most undermines the last part of the passage because it directly contradicts how the law evaluates the use of lethal force. Choices *A* and *B* are stated in the paragraph, so they do not undermine the explanation from the author. Choice *C* does not necessarily undermine the passage, but it does not support the passage either. It is more of an opinion that does not offer strength or weakness to the explanation.

24. C: An assault with deadly intent can lead to an individual using lethal force to preserve their well-being. Choice *C* is correct because it clearly establishes what both assault and lethal force are and gives the specific way in which the two concepts meet. Choice *A* is incorrect because lethal force doesn't necessarily result in assault. This is also why Choice *B* is incorrect. Not all assaults would necessarily be life-threatening to the point where lethal force is needed for self-defense. Choice *D* is compelling but ultimately too vague; the statement touches on aspects of the two ideas but fails to present the concrete way in which the two are connected to each other.

25. A: Both passages open by defining a legal concept and then continue to describe situations in order to further explain the concept. Choice *D* is incorrect because while the passages utilize examples to help explain the concepts discussed, the author doesn't indicate that they are specific court cases. It's also clear that the passages don't open with examples, but instead, they begin by defining the terms addressed in each passage. This eliminates Choice *B,* and ultimately reveals Choice *A* to be the correct answer. Choice *A* accurately outlines the way both passages are structured. Because the passages follow a nearly identical structure, the Choice *C* can easily be ruled out.

26. C: Intent is very important for determining both lethal force and assault; intent is examined in both parties and helps determine the severity of the issue. Choices *A* and *B* are incorrect because it is clear in both passages that intent is a prevailing theme in both lethal force and assault. Choice *D* is compelling, but if a person uses lethal force to defend himself or herself, the intent of the defender is also examined in order to help determine if there was excessive force used. Choice *C* is correct because it states that intent is important for determining both lethal force and assault, and that intent is used to gauge the severity of the issues. Remember, just as lethal force can escalate to excessive use of force, there are different kinds of assault. Intent dictates several different forms of assault.

27. B: The example is used to demonstrate a single example of two different types of assault, then adding in a third type of assault to the example's conclusion. The example mainly provides an instance of "threatening body language" and "provocative language" with the homeowner gesturing threats to his neighbor. It ends the example by adding a third type of assault: physical strikes. This example is used to show the variant nature of assaults. Choice *A* is incorrect because it doesn't mention the "physical strike" assault at the end and is not specific enough. Choice *C* is incorrect because the example does not say anything about the definition of lethal force or how it might be altered. Choice *D* is incorrect, as the example mentions nothing about cause and effect.

28. A: The tone is exasperated. While contemplative is an option because of the inquisitive nature of the text, Choice *A* is correct because the speaker is annoyed by the thought of being included when he felt that the fellow members of his race were being excluded. The speaker is not nonchalant, nor accepting of the circumstances which he describes.

29. C: Choice *C*, *contented*, is the only word that has different meaning. Furthermore, the speaker expresses objection and disdain throughout the entire text.

30. B: The main focus is to address the feelings of exclusion expressed by African Americans after the establishment of the Fourth of July holiday. While the speaker makes biblical references, it is not the main focus of the passage, thus eliminating Choice *A* as an answer. The passage also makes no mention of wealthy landowners and doesn't speak of any positive response to the historical events, so Choices *C* and *D* are not correct.

31: D: Choice *D* is the correct answer because it clearly makes reference to justice being denied.

32: D: It is an example of hyperbole. Choices *A* and *B* are unrelated. Assonance is the repetition of sounds and commonly occurs in poetry. Parallelism refers to two statements that correlate in some manner. Choice *C* is incorrect because amplification normally refers to clarification of meaning by broadening the sentence structure, while hyperbole refers to a phrase or statement that is being exaggerated.

33: C: Display the equivocation of the speaker and those that he represents. Choice *C* is correct because the speaker is clear about his intention and stance throughout the text. Choice *A* could be true, but the words "common text" is arguable. Choice *B* is also partially true, as another group of people affected by slavery are being referenced. However, the speaker is not trying to convince the audience that injustices have been committed, as it is already understood there have been injustices committed. Choice *D* is also close to the correct answer, but it is not the *best* answer choice possible.

34. B: It denotes a period of time. It is apparent that Lincoln is referring to a period of time within the context of the passage because of how the sentence is structured with the word *ago*.

35. C: Lincoln's reference to *the brave men, living and dead, who struggled here,* proves that he is referring to a battlefield. Choices *A* and *B* are incorrect, as a *civil war* is mentioned and not a war with France or a war in the Sahara Desert. Choice *D* is incorrect because it does not make sense to consecrate a President's ground instead of a battlefield ground for soldiers who died during the American Civil War.

36. D: Abraham Lincoln is the former president of the United States, and he references a "civil war" during his address.

37. A: The audience should consider the death of the people that fought in the war as an example and perpetuate the ideals of freedom that the soldiers died fighting for. Lincoln doesn't address any of the topics outlined in Choices *B*, *C*, or *D*. Therefore, Choice *A* is the correct answer.

38. D: Choice *D* is the correct answer because of the repetition of the word *people* at the end of the passage. Choice *A*, *antimetatabole*, is the repetition of words in a succession. Choice *B*, *antiphrasis*, is a form of denial of an assertion in a text. Choice *C*, *anaphora*, is the repetition that occurs at the beginning of sentences.

39. A: Choice *A* is correct because Lincoln's intention was to memorialize the soldiers who had fallen as a result of war as well as celebrate those who had put their lives in danger for the sake of their country. Choices *B* and *D* are incorrect because Lincoln's speech was supposed to foster a sense of pride among the members of the audience while connecting them to the soldiers' experiences.

40. A: The word *patronage* most nearly means *auspices*, which means *protection* or *support*. Choice *B*, *aberration*, means *deformity* and does not make sense within the context of the sentence. Choice *C*, *acerbic,* means *bitter* and also does not make sense in the sentence. Choice *D, adulation*, is a positive word meaning *praise*, and thus does not fit with the word *condescending* in the sentence.

41. D: *Working man* is most closely aligned with Choice *D, bourgeois.* In the context of the speech, the word *bourgeois* means *working* or *middle class.* Choice *A, plebian*, does suggest *common people*; however, this is a term that is specific to ancient Rome. Choice *B, viscount*, is a European title used to describe a specific degree of nobility. Choice *C, entrepreneur*, is a person who operates their own business.

42. C: In the context of the speech, the term *working man* most closely correlates with Choice *C, working man is someone who works for wages among the middle class.* Choice *A* is not mentioned in the passage and is off-topic. Choice *B* may be true in some cases, but it does not reflect the sentiment described for the term *working man* in the passage. Choice *D* may also be arguably true. However, it is not given as a definition but as *acts* of the working man, and the topics of *field, factory,* and *screen* are not mentioned in the passage.

43. D: *Enterprise* most closely means *cause.* Choices *A, B,* and *C* are all related to the term *enterprise.* However, Dickens speaks of a *cause* here, not a company, courage, or a game. *He will stand by such an enterprise* is a call to stand by a cause to enable the working man to have a certain autonomy over his own economic standing. The very first paragraph ends with the statement that the working man *shall . . . have a share in the management of an institution which is designed for his benefit.*

44. B: The speaker's salutation is one from an entertainer to his audience, and uses the friendly language to connect to his audience before a serious speech. Recall in the first paragraph that the speaker is there to "accompany [the audience] . . . through one of my little Christmas books," making him an author there to entertain the crowd with his own writing. The speech preceding the reading is the passage itself, and, as the tone indicates, a serious speech addressing the "working man." Although the passage speaks of employers and employees, the speaker himself is not an employer of the audience, so Choice *A* is incorrect. Choice *C* is also incorrect, as the salutation is not used ironically, but sincerely, as the speech addresses the well-being of the crowd. Choice *D* is incorrect because the speech is not given by a politician, but by a writer.

45: B: Choice *A* is incorrect because that is the speaker's *first* desire, not his second. Choices *C* and *D* are tricky because the language of both of these is mentioned after the word *second.* However, the speaker doesn't get to the second wish until the next sentence. Choices *C* and *D* are merely prepositions preparing for the statement of the main clause, Choice *B,* for the working man to have a say in his institution which is designed for his benefit.

46. D: The use of "I" could have all of the effects for the reader; it could serve to have a "hedging" effect, allow the reader to connect with the author in a more personal way, and cause the reader to empathize more with the egrets. However, it doesn't distance the reader from the text, thus eliminating Choice *D.*

46. C: In lines 6 and 7, it is stated that avarice can prevent a man from being necessitously poor, but too timorous, or fearful, to achieve real wealth. According to the passage, avarice does tend to make a person very wealthy. The passage states that oppression, not avarice, is the consequence of wealth. The passage does not state that avarice drives a person's desire to be wealthy.

47. D: Paine believes that the distinction that is beyond a natural or religious reason is between king and subjects. He states that the distinction between good and bad is made in heaven. The distinction

126

between male and female is natural. He does not mention anything about the distinction between humans and animals.

48. A: The passage states that the Heathens were the first to introduce government by kings into the world. The quiet lives of patriarchs came before the Heathens introduced this type of government. It was Christians, not Heathens, who paid divine honors to living kings. Heathens honored deceased kings. Equal rights of nature are mentioned in the paragraph, but not in relation to the Heathens.

49. B: Paine asserts that a monarchy is against the equal rights of nature, and cites several parts of scripture that also denounce it. He doesn't say it is against the laws of nature. Because he uses scripture to further his argument, it is not despite scripture that he denounces the monarchy. Paine addresses the law by saying the courts also do not support a monarchical government.

50. A: To be *idolatrous* is to worship idols or heroes, in this case, kings. It is not defined as being deceitful. While idolatry is considered a sin, it is an example of a sin, not a synonym for it. Idolatry may have been considered illegal in some cultures, but it is not a definition for the term.

51. A: The essential meaning of the passage is that the Almighty, God, would disapprove of this type of government. While heaven is mentioned, it is done so to suggest that the monarchical government is irreverent, not that heaven isn't promised. God's disapproval is mentioned, not his punishment. The passage refers to the Jewish monarchy, which required both belief in God and kings.

52. C: Gulliver becomes acquainted with the people and practices of his new surroundings. Choice *C* is the correct answer because it most extensively summarizes the entire passage. While Choices *A* and *B* are reasonable possibilities, they reference portions of Gulliver's experiences, not the whole. Choice *D* is incorrect because Gulliver doesn't express repentance or sorrow in this particular passage.

53. A: Principal refers to *chief* or *primary* within the context of this text. Choice *A* is the answer that most closely aligns with this answer. Choices *B* and *D* make reference to a helper or followers while Choice *C* doesn't meet the description of Gulliver from the passage.

54. C: One can reasonably infer that Gulliver is considerably larger than the children who were playing around him because multiple children could fit into his hand. Choice *B* is incorrect because there is no indication of stress in Gulliver's tone. Choices *A* and *D* aren't the best answer because though Gulliver seems fond of his new acquaintances, he didn't travel there with the intentions of meeting new people or to express a definite love for them in this particular portion of the text.

55. C: The emperor made a *definitive decision* to expose Gulliver to their native customs. In this instance, the word *mind* was not related to a vote, question, or cognitive ability.

56. A: Choice *A* is correct. This assertion does *not* support the fact that games are a commonplace event in this culture because it mentions conduct, not games. Choices *B*, *C*, and *D* are incorrect because these do support the fact that games were a commonplace event.

57. B: Choice *B* is the only option that mentions the correlation between physical ability and leadership positions. Choices *A* and *D* are unrelated to physical strength and leadership abilities. Choice *C* does not make a deduction that would lead to the correct answer—it only comments upon the abilities of common townspeople.

58. D: It emphasizes Mr. Utterson's anguish in failing to identify Hyde's whereabouts. Context clues indicate that Choice *D* is correct because the passage provides great detail of Mr. Utterson's feelings about locating Hyde. Choice *A* does not fit because there is no mention of Mr. Lanyon's mental state. Choice *B* is incorrect; although the text does make mention of bells, Choice *B* is not the *best* answer overall. Choice *C* is incorrect because the passage clearly states that Mr. Utterson was determined, not unsure.

59. A: In the city. The word *city* appears in the passage several times, thus establishing the location for the reader.

60. B: It scares children. The passage states that the Juggernaut causes the children to scream. Choices *A* and *D* don't apply because the text doesn't mention either of these instances specifically. Choice *C* is incorrect because there is nothing in the text that mentions space travel.

61. B: To constantly visit. The mention of *morning*, *noon*, and *night* make it clear that the word *haunt* refers to frequent appearances at various locations. Choice *A* doesn't work because the text makes no mention of levitating. Choices *C* and *D* are not correct because the text makes mention of Mr. Utterson's anguish and disheartenment because of his failure to find Hyde but does not make mention of Mr. Utterson's feelings negatively affecting anyone else.

62. D: This is an example of alliteration. Choice *D* is the correct answer because of the repetition of the *L*-words. Hyperbole is an exaggeration, so Choice *A* doesn't work. No comparison is being made, so no simile or metaphor is being used, thus eliminating Choices *B* and *C*.

63. D: The speaker intends to continue to look for Hyde. Choices *A* and *B* are not possible answers because the text doesn't refer to any name changes or an identity crisis, despite Mr. Utterson's extreme obsession with finding Hyde. The text also makes no mention of a mistaken identity when referring to Hyde, so Choice *C* is also incorrect.

64. D: The use of "I" could have all of the effects for the reader; it could serve to have a "hedging" effect, allow the reader to connect with the author in a more personal way, and cause the reader to empathize more with the egrets. However, it doesn't distance the reader from the text, thus eliminating Choice *D*.

65. C: The quote provides an example of a warden protecting one of the colonies. Choice *A* is incorrect because the speaker of the quote is a warden, not a hunter. Choice *B* is incorrect because the quote does not lighten the mood, but shows the danger of the situation between the wardens and the hunters. Choice *D* is incorrect because there is no humor found in the quote.

66. D: A *rookery* is a colony of breeding birds. Although *rookery* could mean Choice *A*, houses in a slum area, it does not make sense in this context. Choices *B* and *C* are both incorrect, as this is not a place for hunters to trade tools or for wardens to trade stories.

67. B: An important bird colony. The previous sentence is describing "twenty colonies" of birds, so what follows should be a bird colony. Choice *A* may be true, but we have no evidence of this in the text. Choice *C* does touch on the tension between the hunters and wardens, but there is no official "Bird Island Battle" mentioned in the text. Choice *D* does not exist in the text.

68. D: To demonstrate the success of the protective work of the Audubon Association. The text mentions several different times how and why the association has been successful and gives examples to back this fact. Choice *A* is incorrect because although the article, in some instances, calls certain people to act, it is not the purpose of the entire passage. There is no way to tell if Choices *B* and *C* are correct, as they are not mentioned in the text.

69. C: To have a better opportunity to hunt the birds. Choice *A* might be true in a general sense, but it is not relevant to the context of the text. Choice *B* is incorrect because the hunters are not studying lines of flight to help wardens, but to hunt birds. Choice *D* is incorrect because nothing in the text mentions that hunters are trying to build homes underneath lines of flight of birds for good luck.

70. A: It introduces certain insects that transition from water to air. Choice *B* is incorrect because although the passage talks about gills, it is not the central idea of the passage. Choices *C* and *D* are incorrect because the passage does not "define" or "invite," but only serves as an introduction to stoneflies, dragonflies, and mayflies and their transition from water to air.

71. C: The act of shedding part or all of the outer shell. Choices *A, B,* and *D* are incorrect.

72. B: The first paragraph serves as a contrast to the second. Notice how the first paragraph goes into detail describing how insects are able to breathe air. The second paragraph acts as a contrast to the first by stating "[i]t is of great interest to find that, nevertheless, a number of insects spend much of their time under water." Watch for transition words such as "nevertheless" to help find what type of passage you're dealing with.

73: C: The stage of preparation in between molting is acted out in the water, while the last stage is in the air. Choices *A, B,* and *D* are all incorrect. *Instars* is the phase between two periods of molting, and the text explains when these transitions occur.

74. C: The author's tone is informative and exhibits interest in the subject of the study. Overall, the author presents us with information on the subject. One moment where personal interest is depicted is when the author states, "It is of great interest to find that, nevertheless, a number of insects spend much of their time under water."

75. C: Their larva can breathe the air dissolved in water through gills of some kind. This is stated in the last paragraph. Choice *A* is incorrect because the text mentions this in a general way at the beginning of the passage concerning "insects as a whole." Choice *B* is incorrect because this is stated of beetles and water-bugs, and not the insects in question. Choice *D* is incorrect because this is the opposite of what the text says of instars.

76. D: To enlighten the audience on the habits of sun-fish and their hatcheries. Choice *A* is incorrect because although the Adirondack region is mentioned in the text, there is no cause or effect relationships between the region and fish hatcheries depicted here. Choice *B* is incorrect because the text does not have an agenda, but rather is meant to inform the audience. Finally, Choice *C* is incorrect because the text says nothing of how sun-fish mate.

77. B: The word *wise* in this passage most closely means *manner*. Choices *A* and *C* are synonyms of *wise*; however, they are not relevant in the context of the text. Choice *D, ignorance,* is opposite of the word *wise*, and is therefore incorrect.

78. A: Fish at the stage of development where they are capable of feeding themselves. Even if the word *fry* isn't immediately known to the reader, the context gives a hint when it says "until the fry are hatched out and are sufficiently large to take charge of themselves."

79. B: The sun-fish builds it with her tail and snout. The text explains this in the second paragraph: "she builds, with her tail and snout, a circular embankment 3 inches in height and 2 thick." Choice *A* is used in the text as a simile.

80. D: To conclude a sequence and add a final detail. The concluding sequence is expressed in the phrase "[t]he mother sun-fish, having now built or provided her 'hatchery.'" The final detail is the way in which the sun-fish guards the "inclosure." Choices *A, B,* and *C* are incorrect.

81. B: Mr. Button's wife is about to have a baby. The passage begins by giving the reader information about traditional birthing situations. Then, we are told that Mr. and Mrs. Button decide to go against tradition to have their baby in a hospital. The next few passages are dedicated to letting the reader know how Mr. Button dresses and goes to the hospital to welcome his new baby. There is a doctor in this excerpt, as Choice *C* indicates, and Mr. Button does put on clothes, as Choice *D* indicates. However, Mr. Button is not going to the doctor's office nor is he about to go shopping for new clothes.

82. A: The tone of the above passage is nervous and excited. We are told in the fourth paragraph that Mr. Button "arose nervously." We also see him running without caution to the doctor to find out about his wife and baby—this indicates his excitement. We also see him stuttering in a nervous yet excited fashion as he asks the doctor if it's a boy or girl. Though the doctor may seem a bit abrupt at the end, indicating a bit of anger or shame, neither of these choices is the overwhelming tone of the entire passage.

83. C: Dedicated. Mr. Button is dedicated to the task before him. Choice *A*, numbed, Choice *B*, chained, and Choice *D*, moved, all could grammatically fit in the sentence. However, they are not synonyms with *consecrated* like Choice *C* is.

84. D: Giving readers a visual picture of what the doctor is doing. The author describes a visual image— the doctor rubbing his hands together—first and foremost. The author may be trying to make a comment about the profession; however, the author does not "explain the detail of the doctor's profession" as Choice *B* suggests.

85. D: To introduce the setting of the story and its characters. We know we are being introduced to the setting because we are given the year in the very first paragraph along with the season: "one day in the summer of 1860." This is a classic structure of an introduction of the setting. We are also getting a long explanation of Mr. Button, what his work is, who is related to him, and what his life is like in the third paragraph.

86. B: "Talk sense!" is an example of an imperative sentence. An imperative sentence gives a command. The doctor is commanding Mr. Button to talk sense. Choice *A* is an example of an exclamatory sentence, which expresses excitement. Choice *C* is an example of an interrogative sentence—these types of sentences ask questions. Choice *D* is an example of a declarative sentence. This means that the character is simply making a statement.

87. C: The point of view is told in third person omniscient. We know this because the story starts out with us knowing something that the character does not know: that her husband has died. Mrs. Mallard eventually comes to know this, but we as readers know this information before it is broken to her. In third person limited, Choice *D*, we would only see and know what Mrs. Mallard herself knew, and we would find out the news of her husband's death when she found out the news, not before.

88. A: The way Mrs. Mallard reacted to her husband's death. The irony in this story is called situational irony, which means the situation that takes place is different than what the audience anticipated. At the beginning of the story, we see Mrs. Mallard react with a burst of grief to her husband's death. However, once she's alone, she begins to contemplate her future and says the word "free" over and over. This is quite a different reaction from Mrs. Mallard than what readers expected from the first of the story.

89. B: The word "elusive" most closely means "indefinable." Horrible, Choice *A*, doesn't quite fit with the tone of the word "subtle" that comes before it. Choice *C*, "quiet," is more closely related to the word "subtle." Choice *D*, "joyful," also doesn't quite fit the context here. "Indefinable" is the best option.

90. D: Mrs. Mallard, a newly widowed woman, finds unexpected relief in her husband's death. A summary is a brief explanation of the main point of a story. The story mostly focuses on Mrs. Mallard and her reaction to her husband's death, especially in the room when she's alone and contemplating the present and future. All of the other answer choices except Choice *C* are briefly mentioned in the story; however, they are not the main focus of the story.

91. D: The interesting thing about this story is that feelings that are confused, joyful, and depressive all play a unique and almost equal part of this story. There is no one right answer here, because the author seems to display all of these emotions through the character of Mrs. Mallard. She displays feelings of depressiveness by her grief at the beginning; then, when she receives feelings of joy, she feels moments of confusion. We as readers cannot help but go through these feelings with the character. Thus, the author creates a tone of depression, joy, and confusion, all in one story.

92. C: The word "tumultuously" most nearly means "violently." Even if you don't know the word "tumultuously," look at the surrounding context to figure it out. The next few sentences we see Mrs. Mallard striving to "beat back" the "thing that was approaching to possess her." We see a fearful and almost violent reaction to the emotion that she's having. Thus, her chest would rise and fall turbulently, or violently.

93. D: To define and describe instances of spinoff technology. This is an example of a purpose question—*why* did the author write this? The article contains facts, definitions, and other objective information without telling a story or arguing an opinion. In this case, the purpose of the article is to inform the reader. The only answer choice that is related to giving information is Choice *D*: to define and describe.

94. A: A general definition followed by more specific examples. This organization question asks readers to analyze the structure of the essay. The topic of the essay is about spinoff technology; the first paragraph gives a general definition of the concept, while the following two paragraphs offer more detailed examples to help illustrate this idea.

95. C: They were looking for ways to add health benefits to food. This reading comprehension question can be answered based on the second paragraph—scientists were concerned about astronauts' nutrition and began researching useful nutritional supplements. Choice *A* in particular is not true because it reverses the order of discovery (first NASA identified algae for astronaut use, and then it was further developed for use in baby food).

96. B: Related to the brain. This vocabulary question could be answered based on the reader's prior knowledge; but even for readers who have never encountered the word "neurological" before, the passage does provide context clues. The very next sentence talks about "this algae's potential to boost brain health," which is a paraphrase of "neurological benefits." From this context, readers should be able to infer that "neurological" is related to the brain.

97. D: To give an example of valuable space equipment. This purpose question requires readers to understand the relevance of the given detail. In this case, the author mentions "costly and crucial equipment" before mentioning space suit visors, which are given as an example of something that is very valuable. Choice *A* is not correct because fashion is only related to sunglasses, not to NASA equipment. Choice *B* can be eliminated because it is simply not mentioned in the passage. While Choice *C* seems like it could be a true statement, it is also not relevant to what is being explained by the author.

98. C: It is difficult to make money from scientific research. The article gives several examples of how businesses have been able to capitalize on NASA research, so it is unlikely that the author would agree with this statement. Evidence for the other answer choices can be found in the article: for Choice *A*, the author mentions that "many consumers are unaware that products they are buying are based on NASA research"; Choice *B* is a general definition of spinoff technology; and Choice *D* is mentioned in the final paragraph.

99. D: The passage does not proceed in chronological order since it begins by pointing out Leif Erikson's explorations in America so Choice *A* does not work. Although the author compares and contrasts Erikson with Christopher Columbus, this is not the main way the information is presented; therefore, Choice *B* does not work. Neither does Choice *C* because there is no mention of or reference to cause and effect in the passage. However, the passage does offer a conclusion (Leif Erikson deserves more credit) and premises (first European to set foot in the New World and first to contact the natives) to substantiate Erikson's historical importance. Thus, Choice *D* is correct.

100. C: Choice *A* is wrong because it describes facts: Leif Erikson was the son of Erik the Red and historians debate Leif's date of birth. These are not opinions. Choice *B* is wrong; that Erikson called the land Vinland is a verifiable fact as is Choice *D* because he did contact the natives almost 500 years before Columbus. Choice *C* is the correct answer because it is the author's opinion that Erikson deserves more credit. That, in fact, is his conclusion in the piece, but another person could argue that Columbus or another explorer deserves more credit for opening up the New World to exploration. Rather than being an incontrovertible fact, it is a subjective value claim.

101. B: Choice *A* is wrong because the author aims to go beyond describing Erikson as a mere legendary Viking. Choice *C* is wrong because the author does not focus on Erikson's motivations, let alone name the spreading of Christianity as his primary objective. Choice *D* is wrong because it is a premise that Erikson contacted the natives 500 years before Columbus, which is simply a part of supporting the author's conclusion. Choice *B* is correct because, as stated in the previous answer, it accurately identifies the author's statement that Erikson deserves more credit than he has received for being the first European to explore the New World.

102. B: Choice *A* is wrong because the author is not in any way trying to entertain the reader. Choice *D* is wrong because he goes beyond a mere suggestion; "suggest" is too vague. Although the author is certainly trying to alert the readers (make them aware) of Leif Erikson's underappreciated and unheralded accomplishments, the nature of the writing does not indicate the author would be satisfied with the reader merely knowing of Erikson's exploration (Choice *C*). Rather, the author would want the reader to be informed about it, which is more substantial (Choice *B*).

103. D: Choice *A* is wrong because the author never addresses the Vikings' state of mind or emotions. Choice *B* is wrong because the author does not elaborate on Erikson's exile and whether he would have become an explorer if not for his banishment. Choice *C* is wrong because there is not enough information to support this premise. It is unclear whether Erikson informed the King of Norway of his finding. Although it is true that the King did not send a follow-up expedition, he could have simply chosen not to expend the resources after receiving Erikson's news. It is not possible to logically infer whether Erikson told him. Choice *D* is correct because there are two examples—Leif Erikson's date of birth and what happened during the encounter with the natives—of historians having trouble pinning down important dates in Viking history.

104. B: But in fact, there is not much substance to such speculation, and most anti-Stratfordian arguments can be refuted with a little background about Shakespeare's time and upbringing. The thesis is a statement that contains the author's topic and main idea. The main purpose of this article is to use historical evidence to provide counterarguments to anti-Stratfordians. Choice *A* is simply a definition; Choice *C* is a supporting detail, not a main idea; and Choice *D* represents an idea of anti-Stratfordians, not the author's opinion.

105. C: Rhetorical question. This requires readers to be familiar with different types of rhetorical devices. A rhetorical question is a question that is asked not to obtain an answer but to encourage readers to consider an issue more deeply.

106. B: By explaining grade school curriculum in Shakespeare's time. This question asks readers to refer to the organizational structure of the article and demonstrate understanding of how the author provides details to support the argument. This particular detail can be found in the second paragraph: "even though he did not attend university, grade school education in Shakespeare's time was actually quite rigorous."

107. A: Busy. This is a vocabulary question that can be answered using context clues. Other sentences in the paragraph describe London as "the most populous city in England" filled with "crowds of people," giving an image of a busy city full of people. Choice *B* is incorrect because London was in Shakespeare's home country, not a foreign one. Choice *C* is not mentioned in the passage. Choice *D* is not a good answer choice because the passage describes how London was a popular and important city, probably not an underdeveloped one.

108. B: This sentence is an example of a metaphor. Metaphors make a comparison between two things, usually saying that one thing *is* another thing. Here, the author is saying that Shakespeare *is* "the great magician." Choice *A*, personification, is when an inanimate object is given human characteristics, so this is incorrect. Choice *C*, simile, is making a comparison between two things using *like* or *as*, so this is incorrect. Choice *D*, allusion, is an indirect reference to a place, person, or event that happened in the past, so this is also incorrect.

109. D: Remember from the first passage that anti-Stratfordians are those who believe that Shakespeare *did not* write the plays, so Stratfordians are people who believe that Shakespeare *did* write the plays. The author of Passage 2 is disbelieving and critical of the Stratfordian point of view. We see this especially in the second paragraph, where the author states it is a supposition "so wild that it can only be entertained by those who are prepared to accept it as a miracle." All of the other answer choices are incorrect.

110. D: Sentence 2 is a contrast to the idea in Sentence 1. In the first sentence, the author states that they, at one time, believed that Shakespeare was the author of his plays. The second sentence is a contrast to that statement by saying the author no longer believes that the author of the plays is Shakespeare. The other answer choices are incorrect.

111. B: This writing style is best described as persuasive. The author is trying to persuade the audience, with evidence, that Shakespeare actually wrote his own dramas. Choice *A*, expository writing, means to inform or explain. Expository writing usually does not set out to persuade the audience of something, only to inform them, so this choice is incorrect. Choice *C*, narrative writing, is used to tell a story, so this is incorrect. Choice *D*, descriptive writing, uses all five senses to paint a picture for the reader, so this choice is also incorrect.

112. C: Topography is the shape and features of the Earth. The author is implying here that whoever wrote Shakespeare's plays studied the physical features of foreign cities. Choices *A, B,* and *D* are incorrect. Choice *A* is simply known as climate. Choice *B* would just be considered the "agriculture of a particular area." Choice *D*, aspects of humans within society, would be known as *anthropology.*

113. A: The author of Passage 2 believes that Shakespeare the actor did not write the plays. We see this at the end of the first paragraph where the author contends that the "'Stratford rustic' is not the true Shakespeare." The author does believe that Shakespeare was an actor, as the author calls this Shakespeare a "Player" throughout the text, so Choices *B* and *D* are incorrect. Choice *C* is incorrect, as the author does not believe that Shakespeare wrote the plays.

114. D: That in order to write about the topography and civilization of a place, one must have travelled there and mingled with the people. We are clear the two authors would disagree over this sentiment. The author of Passage 1 says that "[o]ne needn't travel the continent in order to learn and write about its culture." The author of Passage 2 says "that *he* should have travelled into foreign lands, studied the life and topography of foreign cities" is an assertion that the one who wrote the plays *must have* travelled into foreign lands and studied the life and topography of foreign cities. Choice *A* is something the author of Passage 2 quotes, but we can assume both the authors *do care* whether or not Shakespeare wrote the plays. Choices *B and C* are close. However, the author of Passage 2 does not mention the country education, so we do not know their opinion on Choice *C*. The author does hint that the socioeconomic status of the "rustic" actor would be a limitation to Shakespeare's abilities. However, the author of Passage 2 is most straightforward about Choice *D*.

115. D: This is the argument that the author voices in the second paragraph of Passage 2. A country education and socioeconomic status do not deflect true genius if the individual is willing to absorb the textual and cultural knowledge surrounding them. Choice *A* is incorrect; there is no "new evidence" mentioned in the first passage about Shakespeare having travelled. Choice *B* is incorrect; there is no evidence from Shakespeare's peers that he wrote the plays. Choice *C* is incorrect; this is the author's belief in Passage 2, not Passage 1.

116. B: Passage 1 is written in opposition to Passage 2. We can see the author of Passage 1 stating that it's likely that Shakespeare wrote his own plays. The author of Passage 2 says that it is unlikely that Shakespeare wrote his own plays. This makes Choices *A* and *C* incorrect. Choice *D* is incorrect because we have no direct quotation in Passage 1 that comes directly from Passage 2, only general concepts.

117. A: The last phrase is an example of a rhetorical question. Rhetorical questions are asked in order to make a dramatic effect or point rather than to receive an actual answer. Choice *B*, literary allusion, are indirect references to some historical event, person, or object. Choice *C*, hyperbole, is an exaggeration of something, so this is incorrect. Choice *D*, symbolism, is used to represent an idea or quality of something, like how a rose symbolizes love in western culture.

118. B: Strong dislike. This vocabulary question can be answered using context clues and common sense. Based on the rest of the conversation, the reader can gather that Albert isn't looking forward to his marriage. As the Count notes that "you don't appear to me to be very enthusiastic on the subject of this marriage," and also remarks on Albert's "objection to a young lady who is both rich and beautiful," readers can guess Albert's feelings. The answer choice that most closely matches "objection" and "not . . . very enthusiastic" is *B*, "strong dislike."

119. C: Their name is more respected than the Danglars'. This inference question can be answered by eliminating incorrect answers. Choice *A* is tempting, considering that Albert mentions money as a concern in his marriage. However, although he may not be as rich as his fiancée, his father still has a stable income of 50,000 francs a year. Choice *B* isn't mentioned at all in the passage, so it's impossible to make an inference. Finally, Choice *D* is clearly false because Albert's father arranged his marriage but his mother doesn't approve of it. Evidence for Choice *C* can be found in the Count's comparison of Albert and Eugénie: "she will enrich you, and you will ennoble her." In other words, the Danglars are wealthier but the Morcef family has a more noble background.

120. D: Apprehensive. As in question 7, there are many clues in the passage that indicate Albert's attitude towards his marriage—far from enthusiastic, he has many reservations. This question requires test takers to understand the vocabulary in the answer choices. "Pragmatic" is closest in meaning to "realistic," and "indifferent" means "uninterested." The only word related to feeling worried, uncertain, or unfavorable about the future is "apprehensive."

121. B: He is like a wise uncle, giving practical advice to Albert. Choice *A* is incorrect because the Count's tone is friendly and conversational. Choice *C* is also incorrect because the Count questions why Albert doesn't want to marry a young, beautiful, and rich girl. While the Count asks many questions, he isn't particularly "probing" or "suspicious"—instead, he's asking to find out more about Albert's situation and then give him advice about marriage.

122. A: She belongs to a noble family. Though Albert's mother doesn't appear in the scene, there's more than enough information to answer this question. More than once is his family's noble background mentioned (not to mention that Albert's mother is the Comtess de Morcef, a noble title). The other answer choices can be eliminated—she is obviously deeply concerned about her son's future; money isn't her highest priority because otherwise she would favor a marriage with the wealthy Danglars; and Albert describes her "clear and penetrating judgment," meaning she makes good decisions.

123. C: The richest people in society were also the most respected. The Danglars family is wealthier but the Morcef family has a more aristocratic name, which gives them a higher social standing. Evidence for the other answer choices can be found throughout the passage: Albert mentioned receiving money from his father's fortune after his marriage; Albert's father has arranged this marriage for him; and the Count speculates that Albert's mother disapproves of this marriage because Eugénie isn't from a noble background like the Morcef family, implying that she would prefer a match with a girl from aristocratic society.

124. A: He seems reluctant to marry Eugénie, despite her wealth and beauty. This is a reading comprehension question, and the answer can be found in the following lines: "'I confess,' observed Monte Cristo, 'that I have some difficulty in comprehending your objection to a young lady who is both rich and beautiful.'" Choice *B* is the opposite (Albert's father is the one who insists on the marriage), Choice *C* incorrectly represents Albert's eagerness to marry, and Choice *D* describes a more positive attitude than Albert actually feels ("repugnance").

125. A: First person. This is a straightforward question that requires readers to know that a first-person narrator speaks from an "I" point of view.

126. D: He doesn't understand all of the languages being used. This can be inferred from the fact that the traveler must refer to his dictionary to understand those around him. Choice *A* isn't a good choice because the traveler seems to wonder why the driver needs to drive so fast. Choice *B* isn't mentioned in the passage, and doesn't seem like a good answer choice in the first place because he seems wholly unfamiliar with his surroundings, which is also why Choice *C* can be eliminated.

127. B: From fearful to charmed. This can be found in the first sentence of the third paragraph, which states, "I soon lost sight and recollection of ghostly fears in the beauty of the scene as we drove along." Also, readers should get a sense of foreboding from the first two paragraphs, where superstitious villagers seem frightened on the traveler's behalf. However, the final paragraph changes to delighted descriptions of the landscape's natural beauty. Choices *A* and *D* can be eliminated because the traveler is anxious, not relaxed or comfortable at the beginning of the passage. Choice *C* can also be eliminated because the traveler doesn't gain any particular insights in the last paragraph, and in fact continues to lament that he cannot understand the speech of those around him.

128. D: A complete stranger. The answer to this reading comprehension question can be found in the second paragraph, when the traveler is "just starting for an unknown place to meet an unknown man"—in other words, a complete stranger.

129. C: The traveler will soon encounter danger or evil. Answering this prediction question requires readers to understand foreshadowing, or hints that the author gives about what will happen next. There are numerous hints scattered throughout this passage: the villager's sorrow and sympathy for the traveler and their superstitious actions; the spooky words that the traveler overhears; the driver's unexplained haste. All of these point to a danger that awaits the protagonist.

130. A: "I must say they weren't cheering to me, for amongst them were "Ordog"—Satan, "pokol"—hell, "stregoica"—witch, "vrolok" and "vlkoslak"—both of which mean the same thing, one being Slovak and the other Servian for something that is either were-wolf or vampire." As mentioned in question 39, this sentence is an example of how the author hints at evil to come for the traveler. The other answer choices aren't related to the passage's grim foreshadowing.

131. B: Narrative, Choice *A*, means a written account of connected events. Think of narrative writing as a story. Choice *C*, expository writing, generally seeks to explain or describe some phenomena, whereas Choice *D*, technical writing, includes directions, instructions, and/or explanations. This passage is definitely persuasive writing, which hopes to change someone's beliefs based on an appeal to reason or emotion. The author is aiming to convince the reader that smoking is terrible. They use health, price, and beauty in their argument against smoking, so Choice *B*, persuasive, is the correct answer.

132. B: The author is clearly opposed to tobacco. He cites disease and deaths associated with smoking. He points to the monetary expense and aesthetic costs. Choice *A* is wrong because alternatives to smoking are not even addressed in the passage. Choice *C* is wrong because it does not summarize the passage but rather is just a premise. Choice *D* is wrong because, while these statistics are a premise in the argument, they do not represent a summary of the piece. Choice *B* is the correct answer because it states the three critiques offered against tobacco and expresses the author's conclusion.

133. C: We are looking for something the author would agree with, so it will almost certainly be anti-smoking or an argument in favor of quitting smoking. Choice *A* is wrong because the author does not speak against means of cessation. Choice *B* is wrong because the author does not reference other substances, but does speak of how addictive nicotine, a drug in tobacco, is. Choice *D* is wrong because the author certainly would not encourage reducing taxes to encourage a reduction of smoking costs, thereby helping smokers to continue the habit. Choice *C* is correct because the author is definitely attempting to persuade smokers to quit smoking.

134. D: Here, we are looking for an opinion of the author's rather than a fact or statistic. Choice *A* is wrong because quoting statistics from the Centers of Disease Control and Prevention is stating facts, not opinions. Choice *B* is wrong because it expresses the fact that cigarettes sometimes cost more than a few gallons of gas. It would be an opinion if the author said that cigarettes were not affordable. Choice *C* is incorrect because yellow stains are a known possible adverse effect of smoking. Choice *D* is correct as an opinion because smell is subjective. Some people might like the smell of smoke, they might not have working olfactory senses, and/or some people might not find the smell of smoke akin to "pervasive nastiness," so this is the expression of an opinion. Thus, Choice *D* is the correct answer.

135. C: This is a tricky question, but it can be solved through careful context analysis and vocabulary knowledge. One can infer that the use of "expedient," while not necessarily very positive, isn't inherently bad in this context either. Note how in the next line, he says, "but most governments are usually, and all governments are sometimes, inexpedient." This use of "inexpedient" indicates that a government becomes a hindrance rather than a solution; it slows progress rather than helps facilitate progress. Thus, Choice *A* and Choice *D* can be ruled out because these are more of the result of government, not the intention or initial design. Choice *B* makes no logical sense. Therefore, Choice *C* is the best description of *expedient.* Essentially, Thoreau is saying that government is constructed as a way of developing order and people's rights, but the rigidness of government soon inhibits justice and human rights.

136. B: While Choice *D* is the only answer that mentions the Mexican War directly, Thoreau clearly thinks the war is unnecessary because the people generally didn't consent to the war. Choices *A*, *B*, and *C* are all correct to a degree, but the answer asks for the best description. Therefore, Choice *B* is the most accurate representation of Thoreau's views. Essentially, Thoreau brings to light the fact that the few people in power can twist government and policy for their own needs.

137. D: Choice *C* and Choice *B* are completely incorrect. Thoreau is not defending government in any way. His views are set against government. As mentioned in the text, he appreciates little government but favors having no government structure at all. The text is reflective by nature, but what makes Choice *D* a more appropriate answer is the presence of evidence in the text. Thoreau cites current events and uses them to illustrate the point he's trying to make.

138. C: One of Thoreau's biggest criticisms of government is its capacity to impose on the people's freedoms and liberties, enacting rules that the people don't want and removing power from the individual. None of the scenarios directly impose specific regulations or restrictions on the people, except Prohibition. Prohibition removed the choice to consume alcohol in favor of abstinence, which was favored by the religious conservatives of the time. Thus, Thoreau would point out that this is a clear violation of free choice and an example of government meddling.

139. A: Choice *B* is totally irrelevant. Choice *C* is also incorrect; Thoreau never personifies government. Also, this doesn't coincide with his wooden gun analogy. Choice *D* is compelling because of its language but doesn't define the statement. Choice *A* is the most accurate summary of the main point of Thoreau's statement.

140. B: Thoreau specifically cites that legislators "are continually putting in their way." This reflects his suspicion and concern of government intervention. Recall that Thoreau continually mentions that government, while meant as a way to establish freedom, is easily used to suppress freedom, piling on regulations and rules that inhibit progress. Choice *B* is the answer that most directly states how Thoreau sees government getting in the way of freedom.

141. A: Even though it isn't clear who Boltzmann is, analyzing the content of the passage will reveal clues to what field he most likely studies. While anthropology, the study of humans, might be relevant further into the passage, the writer doesn't open his passage with a specific focus on human origins or studies, so Choice *C* can be eliminated. Choice *D* can also be eliminated because the passage isn't focused on how increasing the food supply would be done—this is presented more as an abstract example. Dietician is a very tempting choice, especially since the article deals with the need for organisms to consume resources for energy, but the correct answer is physicist. Boltzmann was, in fact, a physicist, but even without knowing this fact, there are clues that reveal his field. Note how this text emphasizes the perpetuating relationship between mass and energy. The field of physics is defined as the study of nature as well as the interplay of mass and energy. Choice *A* is correct.

142. C: This is another tricky question that doesn't give the precise answer but instead relies on the careful reading of the text and the knowledge of the reader. Essentially, the passage is discussing how energy consumption is a major factor in evolution and how this can apply to human sustainment and life in general. Living beings must consume food/resources to survive, and the food is converted to energy; energy consumption and conservation are key focuses of survival and evolution—the themes of the text. Organisms must then draw from resources where they live, which is occupied by other organisms. Therefore, in this case, competing doesn't necessarily refer to combat but to the fact that many organisms are trying to survive off the same or similar resources simultaneously. Essentially, they are coexisting together and struggling to live off the land. Choice *C* is the best choice.

143. D: Choice *A* is very tempting; it's clear that his goal is to educate the reader on a concept within evolution. Choice *B* is totally incorrect. Energy clearly does have an impact on evolution. Choice *C* is also compelling. The author does use an example of how environmental shifts can impact the population; he hasn't yet proposed a plan of study or urged the reader to support a specific environmental enhancement study. Choice *D* is actually very similar to Choice *A*. What makes Choice *D* the optimal answer is the specific use of capturing energy, which is more consistent with the text. The author also elaborates on how energy impacts evolution and the survival of key traits. He is educating the reader, but he's also trying to prove his point about energy and evolution.

144. B: Choice *A* can be immediately eliminated, as the passage specifically states, "whenever such organisms arise, natural selection will operate to preserve and increase them." This literally means that these positive traits will be passed on to following generations, increasing their chances of survival within the flux of the natural world. Choices *C* and *D* are incorrect for similar reasons.

145. D: Choice *B* is clearly incorrect because the author goes into detail about how the three concepts are interconnected. On that note, Choice *A* is somewhat backward, as evolution is not a constant but a resulting trend. Energy does not create evolution, nor does evolution necessarily create shifting mass amounts. Rather, evolution occurs through a result of several key factors such as energy influencing the mass of an organism and the organism's successful use of that stored energy. Thus, Choice *D* is the accurate summary. Choice *C* is incorrect because no rate of evolution is mentioned specifically.

146. C: Note the language in this quote and the paragraph it belongs to. In this scenario, mass is not being increased to develop more energy. Rather, the increase of energy/velocity would boost the impact of the mass life cycle. Mass becomes more productive and expels more work through the boost in energy. Choice *A* is an example of mass being increased, resulting in increased energy, not what this section is referring to. Choices B and D are irrelevant; they really don't deal with matter and energy. Choice C, however, matches very well with the quote. While the water (matter) does not increase, the velocity of the water increases, which enables more energy to be gained from the mill.

147. A: Choice D can be eliminated because the Salem witch trials aren't even mentioned. While sympathetic to the plight of the accused, the author doesn't demand or urge the reader to demand reparations to the descendants; therefore, Choice B can also be ruled out. It's clear that the author's main goal is to educate the reader and shed light on the facts and hidden details behind the case. However, his focus isn't on the occult, but the specific Lancashire case itself. He goes into detail about suspects' histories and ties to Catholicism, revealing how the fears of the English people at the time sealed the fate of the accused witches. Choice A is correct.

148. B: It's important to note that these terms may not be an exact analog for *enduring*. However, through knowledge of the definition of *enduring*, as well as the context in which it's used, an appropriate synonym can be found. Plugging "circumstantial" into the passage in place of "enduring" doesn't make sense. Nor does "un-original," this particular case of witchcraft, stand out in history. "Wicked" is very descriptive, but this is an attribute applied to people, not events; therefore, this is an inappropriate choice as well. *Enduring* literally means long lasting, referring to the continued interest in this particular case of witchcraft. Therefore, it's a popular topic of 1600s witch trials, making "popular," Choice B, the best choice.

149. D: Choices A and B are irrelevant and clearly incorrect. The use of quotes truly does lend some credibility to the author, especially if applied well, which this author does. However, the presence of quotes alone doesn't necessarily mean that the author has a qualified perspective. What really establishes the writer as a reliable voice is the fact that he has not only researched the material but has had his previous writing on the subject published before. The author's insight and historical knowledge are clearly valued and respected enough for him to have achieved publications. This qualification greatly establishes his credentials as a historical writer, making Choice D the answer.

150. B: Choice A is incorrect, clearly taking the statement somewhat literally. The remaining three choices appear somewhat interconnected, and though they may be proven at some point later in the article, the focus must remain on the given excerpt. It's very possible that evidence was tampered with or even falsified, but this statement doesn't refer to this. While the author alludes that there may have been evidence tampering and potentially corruption, what the writer is directly saying is that the documentation of the court indicates an elaborate trial. It's clear that exaggerations may have taken place both during the case and in the written account. The reasoning behind this was to gain the attention of the people and even the crown. Choice B is the best answer because it not only aligns with the above statement, but ultimately encompasses the potentiality of Choices C and D as well.

151. C: Conceivably, several of these answers could have contributed to the fear and political motivations around the Lancashire witch trials. What this answer's looking for is very specific: political motivations and issues that played a major role in the case. Political, of course, means relating to government or public affairs. Choice D can be eliminated; while this information may have some truth and is certainly consistent with the general fear of witchcraft, the details about Lancashire's ancient history aren't mentioned in the text. Choice A is certainly true but not necessarily political in nature. Choice B is very promising, though not outright mentioned. Choice C clearly outlines the public fears of the time. It also describes how the government can use this fear to weed out and eliminate traces of Catholicism (and witchcraft too). Catholicism and witchcraft were seen as dangerous and undermining to English Protestantism and governance. Choice C is the best answer.

152. D: Choice *B* can be immediately ruled out; spectral evidence isn't mentioned. The evidence of the case draws on knowledge of superstition of witchcraft, but this in itself can't be considered evidence. Choice *A* is incorrect. Choice *C* isn't really evidence in a modern or practical sense; rumors have no weight in court and therefore are not evidence. While this is used as evidence to some degree, this still isn't the *best* evidence against Alizon and the witches. In fact, the best evidence comes from Alizon herself. The text mentions that she confessed to bewitching John Law, thinking that she actually did him harm. From here she names her grandmother, who she believes corrupted her—this is where popular rumors and suspicion of witchcraft and Catholicism come into play. However, it began with the initial self-incriminating speech that opened the doors for the rest of the case to happen. Choice *D* is correct.

153. D: If unfamiliar with this term, plugging each term into the sentence in place of "elucidation" will help rule out answers that don't make sense. Using this method, Choices *B* and *C* can be ruled out because they don't fit the sentence. "Definition" looks promising, but this term isn't as comprehensive an explanation. After all, the author is seeking to uncover why myths are the way they are—the reason why there are so many shared concepts. "Rank" is looking for an explanation for why myths appear as they do. In fact, *explanation* is a synonym for *elucidation*. Choice *D* is correct.

154. B: The title and general focus of the passage reveal a lot about the motivations and interests of the writer. This is a study in psychology, so the author's main area of interest is the study of how humans think and process the world. Choice *A* can be eliminated easily. While Rank was in fact a contemporary of Jung, this information is neither relevant nor even mentioned in the text. The other answers are very compelling, but in this case, one must look at what the author already sees in mythology. The reach and similarities in various mythologies suggest a common source—a common humanity. While he doesn't explicitly want to use this knowledge to develop new analysis strategies and therapies (Choice *D*), this does seem to hint to a common human mind-set that would be crucial for his work. Thus, Choice *B* is the best answer. Also, Choice *C* is too narrow and of less interest to the author.

155. A: The key to understanding this theory lies in "the existence of elemental ideas, so that the unanimity of the myths is a necessary sequence of the uniform disposition of the human mind and the manner of its manifestation." In other words, elemental ideas are core questions or ideas that apply to everyone. Choice *B* is compelling, but the idea of winter, and cold climate, doesn't necessarily apply to cultures in climates with mild winters, like in Africa. Choice *C* doesn't offer a lot to consider. Choice *D* is focused on Germanic and Nordic peoples. The best answer will address overarching ideas and concepts that exist throughout the world cultures: elemental ideas. The idea that best exemplifies the Idea of the People theory is Choice *A* because it hints to innate human curiosity and the drive to define the world. Choice *C* can then be ruled out entirely.

156. C: Choice *A* is incorrect; these are not scientific explanations. Choice *B* is incorrect; these are appropriately labeled as "theories, and there is a reason behind this choice. Choice *D* is incorrect and actually a major clue. The author doesn't say that these are competing ideas; rather, he directly says they don't conflict. In truth, all these theories could have a basis in historical fact. However, these can't be proven by physical means. It would be virtually impossible to track, and therefore prove, the exact reason why mythology resonates throughout various cultures and its exact origin. There simply isn't physical evidence. Therefore, these ideas are called *theories* because, while they hold probable truth, they cannot be tested or proven. Choice *C* is correct.

157. D: This can be a very deceptive description, even pessimistic sounding if not considered with the context of the rest of the passage. Choice *A* is incorrect; this takes too rigid a stance on the lines. The quote doesn't condemn people to unoriginality, merely that ideas can be used over and over again, even adapted or copied. Choice *B* looks compelling but doesn't take the rest of the reading into account. Choice *C* is very tempting; it uses similar language to the selection, but note the use of "sundered." Nowhere in the text (both the main passage and the selected quote) is there a mention of sundering or a breakaway from a single culture, but rather the spreading and sharing of ideas. Again, there is also this hint of a lack of originality that isn't necessarily true. Choice *D*, however, is a phrase that perfectly ties the presented quote with the rest of the passage, a kind of bridge that adds another layer to mythology's origins.

158. B: Choice *A* is compelling, but this statement relates more to the migration theory of spreading mythology. It's a little too broad and less focused on community relations. Choice *D* is compelling and might be the best answer without the presence of Choice *B*. Choice *B* clearly displays what the "explanation by original community idea" focuses on. Note how this theory is centered on a central community (or communities) that expands into different areas. Another key point is that the stories "continued to grow while retaining the common primary traits." In other words, the stories might have grown or changed in some ways, but they still retained core aspects in the narrative. This theory is best exemplified in Choice *B*.

159.B: The author specifically states that the use of objects or tools (extraneous substances) by animals is imitative and not done without human influence. The focus here is on the use of objects to advance an independent desire. Discerning this, Choices *A* and *D* can be eliminated; these do not involve tools or objects. This leaves Choices *B* and *C*. Looking closely at Choice *C*, it's clear that while the monkey used an object, and even used it correctly, this action was done mimicking the human in the video, which makes this answer incorrect. Choice *B*, however, is correct. The fact that wild animals use tools without contact with humans means that they did this independent of human influence and instruction.

160. A: While not defining the term, the author provides a lot of context with which to piece together the meaning of *quadrumana*. From the quotes, it's clear that primates are being discussed. Specifically, the term will indicate their ability to hold on to things. With this in mind, common sense/knowledge comes into play. The first part of the word is very recognizable: "quad." This, of course, is the Latin root for *four*. Another Latin root in the term is *mana*, which refers to hands—think of the term *manual*. Together, the word literally means "four-handed," which makes sense because the text deals with animals that have the potential to hold and manipulate substances. Choice *A* is correct.

161. C: This tricky answer can have a couple of different meanings, which can be lost in the complicated writing style the author uses. In the second paragraph, Thompson writes: "We must conclude, further, that the use of tools and weapons, even preceding the intelligent conformation of them for definite purposes, marked the differentiation of primitive man from the animal branch, and accompanied indeed was the cause of the psychic emergence." Here, the author states clearly that the use of tools and weapons came before the actual use of the objects for intelligent and definite purposes. This is a major clue. The author follows up this statement with: "The moment that the primitive man-ape employed extraneous substances intelligently, with a purpose, he ceased to be an ape and became a man. We must believe that the use of tools and the psychic emergence were coincident and interdependent." This statement puts the psychic emergence on a similar level but not necessarily congruent with free will. This was the consciousness of the possibility of shaping reality that enabled humans to choose what to do. Knowing this, some answers can be easily eliminated. Choices *A* and *B* can be ruled out because their contents aren't addressed at all. Choices *C* and *D* are very close, but remember what was just examined: The psychic emergence isn't necessarily free will, but the ability to process the possibility of using natural resources. Thus, choice *C* is the best answer.

162. B: Before going to the answers, it's important to consider what the original quote means. The original translation of *cogito ergo sum* is "I think; therefore, I am." The author modifies this translation to "I think; therefore I exist." Both translations refer to the ability to self-identify. Essentially, because people can think, they can define their own being and can alter themselves to become what they want. The fact that people know they exist means in fact they exist in the world. To answer this question, consider how this relates to the use of tools/weapons. The author argues that when our ape ancestors began using resources, they then began to develop uses and designs to advance their own survival. This in turn established their self-awareness and led to higher cognition. The answer here that best combines both ideas is Choice *B*.

163. D: A scepter is a physical object or ornament that symbolizes both sovereignty and authority; it's a literal object that symbolizes power. The author is saying that the tool itself was the device from which man was able to become independent and shape nature to their advantage. With this in mind, it's clear that Choice *D* correctly captures this clever use of symbolism and relates it back to the whole text.

164. A: Choice *B* was heavily hinted at in the beginning of the fourth paragraph. Recall that the ape was surrounded by dangers; its survival necessitated that it find a way to counter the various threats it faced. While not mentioned in this selection of the text, Choices *C* and *D* seem to parallel Choice *B*. Utilizing its grasping hands to increase its chance for gaining food is a major advantage in survival. Choice *A* clearly stands apart for the simple reason that this situation does not rely on the ape actually using resources in the ways for tools. It's true that the ape is taking advantage of a natural resource, but the ape doesn't seem to create a shelter. The answer details that the apes will seek more caves for protection. This is something modern animals such as bears do to this day. Seeking shelter isn't the same as using devices to manufacture a shelter. Therefore, this example isn't a likely circumstance that would have prompted tool use. Choice *A* is the answer.

165. C: It's very clear that the author is chronicling the development of museums, but is there a defined viewpoint that he is trying to impress upon the reader? No. The author presents facts, and even inferences, but he is clearly not trying to claim something new. Instead, he's simply providing details about the rise of museums by describing the first examples of people collecting and displaying items. This makes Choice *A* and Choice *D* incorrect. Also, the 1850s weren't even mentioned in this excerpt. The author doesn't insert himself into the piece; there's no use of "I." There also isn't any mention of his own experiences. This also means that Choice *B* is incorrect. Clearly, the author is documenting the development of museums by focusing on collections that, while not conforming to modern museums, would give rise to the idea later on. Choice *C* is correct.

166. B: Generally, all the questions seem to hold some truth, but the goal is to find the answer that best explains the excerpt. Choice *C* can be eliminated first. It doesn't address the statement directly; besides, there are traveling exhibits. Choice *D* is very true, but this doesn't provide the reasoning behind the statement. Choice *A* is very strong, but Choice *B* is actually stronger. Choice *B* addresses the fact that a stable society enables the museum to be maintained and visitors to actively visit the museum. Thus, Choice *B* is correct.

167. D: Recall that the text illustrates that initially it was primarily royalty that owned collections and displayed them, but this didn't necessarily mean that these artifacts made up a museum. This eliminates Choice *A*. The author goes on to reflect on how the great institute of Alexandria wouldn't really be considered a museum because "the name museum in that institution was applied to a portion set apart for the study of sciences, and indicated rather a place of study than one for exhibition of objects." While a museum is a place of study, it's clear that the modern museum is primarily geared for exhibition. With this in mind, Choice *B* simply falls short and can be eliminated. The answer that sums up the core criteria for a modern museum is Choice *D*. The purpose of a modern museum is not just to house artifacts but to display them for the public. With this in mind, Choice *C* falls short by not addressing the core role of a museum.

168. A: Choice *C* can be eliminated first; this answer makes no sense. The term "virtues" is modified by "preservative." In other words, the phrase "preservative virtues" is talking about a substance's potential to provide preservation. Preservation is not an act of correction; this doesn't make sense, so Choice *B* can be eliminated. Choice *D* is very promising, but "virtues" isn't referring to the capability of a substance but rather the good qualities within the alcohol. In this case, "virtues" is used as a noun that means specific qualities. Therefore, the most accurate alternative would be "properties," Choice *A*. *Properties* is a noun that means distinctive attributes or qualities.

169. C: Avoid choosing answers that seem exaggerated or subjective. It's well known that Aristotle is an accomplished philosopher and natural history researcher, but this passage doesn't quantify his expertise. While we can infer that Aristotle is highly adept to be highly favored by Alexander, Choice *A* is an opinion that isn't directly stated. Choice *B* may be true, but this is too broad to gauge from this single excerpt. Choice *D* could be possible, but note how Alexander is gathering the material for Aristotle; the text doesn't hint to additional motives for a museum. The best answer is Choice *C*; if Aristotle has an interest in, or at least intends to study natural artifacts, it stands to reason that others may be actively researching natural history.

170. B: Referring back to the essay, it's clear that this information would fit the best in the fourth paragraph. This is where natural curiosities are first mentioned. However, it introduces the idea of misidentifying the natural curiosities too soon and does not allow the author to actually introduce the natural curiosities and their significance. Inserting this information before the final sentence allows the reader to read about actual examples of ancient natural oddities. This new information would then enable the readers to have a full-circle understanding of the items, showing first ancient interpretations and then modern revelations. Choice *B* is the best answer.

171. C: The author is not a geologist, and while there could be physical evidence in the ancient soil levels, he does not bring this information into this section of the passage. Choice *A* is incorrect. The author quotes several contemporary sources who have done research on this topic, but they are also basing their research on ancient accounts/sources. These sources can best be described as textual evidence from the Romans themselves. Note how the author cites specific numbers and historical events that contributed to grain shortage and agricultural decline. This information must have been documented at some point in order to reach modern readers. Therefore, Choice *C* is the best description of actual evidence in the text.

172. A: The passage doesn't mention military attack from barbarians, making Choice *D* irrelevant. Choice *C* is vague and doesn't tie back into agricultural decline. The author argues that Rome fell from within, not that its civilization was destroyed. It makes sense that being unable to produce sufficient food in Italy, Rome would have had to rely on other territories for food. This would have taxed Rome greatly and contributed to economic and even political hardships. Choice *B* is a good choice. Poverty, which was mentioned in the text, became more widespread, which also taxed state granaries. This in itself would have made Rome more dependent on external food sources, but essentially a scenario like Choice *B* mentions would be included in Choice *A*'s scenario. Choice *A* more effectively sums up the result of agricultural decline.

173. D: The main point of Rodbertus' stance is that the agricultural decline had less to do with physical circumstances and more to do with social causes. Therefore, the best evidence in favor of this would be details on how the Roman people themselves or the government affected agriculture. Choice *A* is incorrect because this is a natural occurrence. Choice *C* is compelling; this certainly supports Rodbertus' assertion that Romans were keen agriculturalists. Choice *B* is definitely a good option, but just because many farmers left Rome to pursue farming abroad doesn't necessarily mean agriculture suffered an irreparable blow. Choice *D* is the strongest answer. Note how this answer opens with the idea of taxes creating troubles for farmers. Taxes, of course, are instituted by a social structure: the government. The taxes then made farming difficult by placing strains on the farmers which, as a result, led them to overwork the land to a point that crop yields might have been less productive. This illustrates the trickling sequence of social changes and institutions marring agriculture, which is exactly what Rodbertus believes happened. Therefore, Choice *D* is a stronger answer than Choice *C*. Another consideration: Technology and good practice can only go so far when such resources may be limited by external factors such as policy or regulation.

174. B: The author clearly has a specific idea that he's trying to discuss and prove true to the reader. This makes Choice *C* an incorrect answer. Choice *D* is incorrect as well. The opposing information is not easily dismissed; in fact, the author acknowledges that there appears to be validity in some of the other scholars' observations. However, this doesn't weaken the author's argument. By addressing alternative views, the author is providing a greater context of how the evidence can be interpreted. The use of opposing sources actually strengthens his argumentative style because he has the opportunity to illustrate how others might have been overlooked or incorrectly assessed the information regarding agricultural decline. He goes on to assert this through supplementary sources that favor his ideas. Therefore, Choice *B* is correct.

175. A: close reading of this excerpt is essential here. The author mentions: "Such exhaustion, as he says, is not a necessary consequence of incorrect cultivation, but arises only when unwise methods are pursued." In other words, the technique of collecting crops wasn't flawed, but the methodology might have been poor. This doesn't necessarily mean the Romans were unskilled at farming; perhaps hard times forced them to take unwise steps. Again, Choice *C* is an example of an overexaggeration, which can usually be eliminated in answer options. Choice *B* is incorrect; the passage gives no indication that Rodbertus' observations focused on an irrelevant time period, but rather that he draws from an earlier period than the fall of Rome. This is actually important for people studying agricultural decline to study agriculture over history; earlier agricultural cycles can reveal important trends in the earth and even political atmosphere. Choice *D* is incorrect; the passage gives no indication that soil exhaustion is instantaneous. If anything, the excerpt hints that it may occur over time. Recall the following: "Rodbertus indicates the condition in the early days, when Rome was in her prime. The other presents the conditions of later times." Rodbertus never said there wasn't a time of agricultural decline, but that it might have been the result of social reasons. The second sentence refers to another of Simkhovitch's stance, which reflects a *later period*. This suggests that there was an agricultural decline earlier in history and a separate one that caused the fall of Rome. This in itself hints to other trends of agricultural decay, until a period so bad occurred that it contributed to the demise of Rome. Choice *A* is correct.

176. C: The key to answering this question is to simply summarize the facts in a way that presents a clear quantifiable statement—one that shows measurable effect. The best summary will contain the three main facts. The closest answers to this are Choices *B* and *C*. However, Choice *B* mentions that Romans became dependent on other food sources. The passage doesn't mention this. Also, if the Romans did find an alternative food source, this could have resolved or elevated the agricultural decline to where it wasn't a major cause of the collapsing empire. Choice *C*, however, is far more decisive and comprehensive. Note how this option brings up the consistent decline of farmland and goes further by drawing the connection to its impact on Roman culture, with the passing of laws to restrict serfs to land. This not only shows physical degradation but also highlights the concern of the Roman government about this disturbing trend. Thus, Choice *C* is the best answer.

177. D: The author immediately states that the text is inherently a pagan work with Christian "coloring" applied to make the text appeal to Christian audiences. He acknowledges outright that there are several theories about the origins and original composition of *Beowulf,* but he doesn't state which theory he personally supports (at least, not in this excerpt). Rather, the author acknowledges the views and specifically states: "In the nature of the case we can look for no entire consensus of opinion and no exact answer to the question; the most that one can expect to establish is at the best only a probability." This indicates that he doesn't think a definitive answer can be found, but the theories presented are the most likely that explain *Beowulf*'s origins. The author is merely writing about the potential origins of *Beowulf* and detailing which aspects of the text reflect certain elements of the debate. Therefore, Choice *D* is the best answer.

178. B: The author doesn't seem to have a particular audience, but it's clear from his tone and diction that he means for this work to be read by fellow scholars or advanced students, not children. Choice *A* is incorrect. Choice *D* is also a stretch; remember that the author, while clearly fond of the text, doesn't go into the imagery or artistry of the text. He focuses on how the language could reveal the origins of *Beowulf*. Therefore, Choice *D* is very unlikely. While there are clearly Christian elements in the text of *Beowulf,* the pagan aspects were not completely covered up, which the author clearly acknowledges. Choice *C* is incorrect. Choice *B* is the best answer because this references how the later Christian elements were "colored" into the original myth. Also, the author himself says: "The purpose of the present study is to contribute to the settlement of the question inferences drawn from a careful examination of the passages that show a Christian coloring."

179. A: The author is clearly open-minded and diplomatic in assessing where Christianity is inserted into the *Beowulf* text. Just as with mythology itself, humans have shared values. Things such as loyalty, truth, and defending the weak tend to be heavily valued, just as stealing and murder are frowned upon. The author's acknowledgment of this, and given the fact that the text is based on an original pagan story, it's clear that Christians and pagans did have common moral principles. Choice *A* is correct.

180. C: Choice *A* can be eliminated first; this answer is very vague and unspecific. Choice *B* is compelling but offers no clear evidence that the pagan storyteller even told the story of Beowulf or that it was told/sung in poetical format. Choices *C* and *D* are both very compelling. However, Choice *C* would be the stronger evidence. If there was an account of a monk listening to *Beowulf,* this would be strong evidence for the second theory, but this still doesn't tell of the style of the tale. This situation also wouldn't account for how the Christian monk took the original *Beowulf* poem and compiled it. Choice *C* provides the actual evidence of a monk writing down *Beowulf* lays and trying to organize them into what would become the epic. Therefore, Choice *C* is the best answer.

181. B: This is another situation in which many answers are right, but one is the most right. Choice *A* can be eliminated first; this is a generalization and not true. In reality, Christianity demonized the pagan faiths to garner conversions. The remaining three choices each bear merit and serve as likely motivations for the writer to smear heathen ideas and worship. However, Choice *B* is the most detailed and logical answer.

182. D: Choice *B* is possible but unlikely. Blackburn points out that the writer of *Beowulf* seemed to be knowledgeable of language. Wyrd is not a concept of Christianity. In Christianity, God controls everything. It's unlikely that the author would have thought fate is a major Christian concept, which makes Choice *A* incorrect. Choice *C* is possible but unlikely; it is quite a stretch to assume the author thought fate could be linked to damnation or serve as a warning to behave like Christians. Choice *D* presents the strongest case of all the answers. It is likely that the writer of Beowulf wasn't fully clear on fate and didn't care; after all, he thought paganism was inferior to Christianity. As mentioned, the use of "fate" probably would have also allowed the author to color in a Christianized interpretation of fate, or at least leave "fate" in the text and add Christian symbols around mentions of fate. Thus, Choice *D* is the best answer.

183. A: Choice *D* can be eliminated; the author's discussion indicates there are ways to identify how dinosaurs moved. Choice *C* is incorrect for a similar reason. Choices *A* and *B* are similar, but note how Choice *B* focuses on the debate of how to classify dinosaurs themselves. While this was a debate, this wasn't the focus of this passage. The passage primarily argues on how dinosaurs move and stand in relation to their reptilian qualities; it seems like scientists are debating if dinosaurs should be even considered reptiles. Therefore, Choice *A* is the best answer.

184. B: This is a very tricky question that requires thorough analysis of the context in which it is used. This term is describing the movement patterns of modern elephants and how this likely reflects the movements of *Diplodocus*. One must ask: Which best describes how elephants move their legs and stand? The simple answer is that they stand straight and move their legs in a forward motion. Choices *C* and *D* clearly don't relate. Choice *A* sounds compelling, but elephants, or other large mammals, don't move rectangularly. Thus, Choice *B* is correct; *rectigrade* actually means moving in a straight line.

185. D: While scientists believe dinosaurs were warm-blooded today, this idea isn't even touched upon here. There's no way to gauge what the author would think on this topic, so Choice *A* can be eliminated. Just because the author finds a similarity between elephants and a dinosaur, it's an exaggeration to say that all large animals share movement patterns. Therefore, Choice *D* is incorrect. Choice *B* is incorrect as well. Recall that the author previously mentioned the idea of dinosaurs being reptiles, "yet they form a group apart," in the second paragraph. In other words, while they may be considered reptiles, the author is open to the idea of dinosaurs being a different variation of reptiles not bound by modern reptilian features. Therefore, Choice *D* makes the most sense.

186. B: Conceivably, this information could fit into several areas of the text. The best way to present this new information would be to follow the flow of the essay and not upset the original structure. The information should not disrupt interconnected paragraphs, which would be the case in Choice *D*. This choice would insert the new information randomly between the comparison of the views of key scientists that's crucial for the text. This information put after the second paragraph would disrupt the essay and confuse the reader. Choice *C* would present the same conundrum, though perhaps less so. Choice *A* is a strategy has been applied successfully before by many writers and is not a bad choice, but note how well the writer originally outlines the debate of *Sauropodous* stance and movement from the beginning. He presents a question and then uses the essay to explore it and try to answer the question. Presenting evidence first would ultimately mar the writer's setup. The optimal section for this new information would be at the end of this selection. It would make sense that after discussing bone structure for some time, introducing evidence like footprints next would be very strategic and flow nicely with the essay. Note also how the end of this selection states: "For among mammals there are both straight and curved femora, and a wide variety of gaits." "Gait" refers to walking. Evidence of walking and how a gait can be measured would be best explored by footprint patterns. Thus, Choice *B* is the answer.

187. C. Choice *A* is obviously incorrect. Choice *D* is a very broad assumption and one not based on this information. The author isn't focusing on all dinosaurs; he isn't linking the general movements of the species to that of mammals but merely comprehending how *Diplodocus* might have moved like a mammal. Choice *B* could be true, but the information presented doesn't directly link *Diplodocus* with a variety of gaits. The best answer is Choice *C*. This excerpt clearly relates that the shape of the femur can vary and produce different types of movement—there are other factors in addition to the femur shape that determine an animal's motion.

188. D: This is a little bit of a trick question. The author doesn't state explicitly his views on *Sauropodous* movement/stance, but it's clear that he disagrees that they moved and were structured like modern reptiles. With this in mind, Choices *B* and *C* can be ruled out, as these individuals take stances more in favor of viewing the dinosaurs as having reptilian mechanics. Choice *A* is somewhat compelling, but recall how he explicitly states that "Dr. Hay misstates the supposed significance of the peculiar type of femur seen in Diplodocus." Therefore, there is a bias; he clearly doesn't agree with the views of Hay and Tornier. While the author may not totally agree with Dr. Abel and Dr. Holland, the language does suggest that he agrees with their views. Therefore, Choice *D* is the best answer.

189. C: The author clearly doesn't believe that beliefs or wishes are real in the physical sense. What he's saying here is that these concepts are real and have a transcendental significance in the fact that human cognition gives these meaning. People strive to see or shape the world according to beliefs and wishes. However, according to the writer, these concepts don't come from a higher source and aren't preexisting. According to the author, humans develop and subscribe to dreams and wishes based on the way their experiences have led them to see the world. Therefore, Choice *C* is the closest, best answer.

190. A: Choice *D* is incorrect; the author doesn't state or imply this in the passage. Based on the text, it's possible the author believes there is no free will, but it's not the focus of this essay. Therefore, eliminate Choice *B*. Choice *C* is a very strong answer, but the author's reasoning behind there being no natural law is the fact that essentially every idea and law is subjective. There's no natural law because people choose to act and believe according to their own desires and predispositions. Therefore, natural law doesn't hold ideals/standards that are inherent needs for the quality of human life. Choice *A* really captures the writer's argument.

191. C: All of these answers could be used to counter the author's argument, but one must be fully aware of how the author's argument is structured. The author is saying that natural law doesn't exist, and he is arguing this on two primary levels. The first is that thoughts and beliefs are inherently subjective. The second is that there seems to be no binding necessity that compels or even inspires people to follow natural law. The answer that most directly counters his argument is the one that highlights that this argument is inherently an opinion. Point of fact: The author doesn't use hard evidence, but his interpretation of human nature. These are his views, which are subjective to him, the author's unique viewpoint. This viewpoint, however, cannot be used to dictate that of others, certainly not on a more global scale. It's just his opinion. Therefore, by addressing this, a major blow is struck to the author's argument through his own reasoning. Choice *C* is the best answer and strongest counterargument.

192. D: Choice *A* is clearly an incorrect exaggeration. While Choice *C* is very compelling, it is highly circumstantial. The author is more concerned about the moral implications of the decision than what

147

happened in the end. Therefore, Choice *C* can be ruled out. The first part of Choice *B* appears to be correct, but the second half inherently goes against this. Natural law should apply to a case like the one the author is proving, or at least he thinks that if natural law exists, this case should apply. Choice *B* is close but falls short of focusing on how the writer might have overlooked the situation. The best answer is Choice *D*. The situation could have been dire. The action of closing the hatch might have saved more individuals than trying to save the few in the cargo. The author doesn't consider this information and even acknowledges it with: "It is idle to illustrate further, because to those who agree with me I am uttering commonplaces and to those who disagree I am ignoring the necessary foundations of thought."

193. B: While it's clear that the author doesn't believe the concept of natural law exists, this doesn't mean he thinks law has no utility. Choice *A* is incorrect. Choice *C* is possible; he does reference a legal case, but he doesn't use specific legal terms or cite other cases to prove his point. There is not enough information in this selection to infer whether he is or isn't a defense lawyer. With this logic, Choice *C* can be ruled out. Choice *D* is probably true, but for this question, the answer will be one that draws from information directly in the text. The author doesn't discuss human reasoning or existence as a species. Choice *D* is incorrect. Choice *B* is the best answer. Clearly, the author believes that predisposition influences what people want, believe, and aspire to do. He likely doesn't think that we are born with our nature already set. Rather, exterior forces, such as upbringing, make us who we are. Consider this quote from the text as evidence: "But I do agree with them in believing that one's attitude on these matters is closely connected with one's general attitude toward the universe. Proximately, as has been suggested, it is determined largely by early associations and temperament, coupled with the desire to have an absolute guide." Note the emphasis on "early associations" influencing the person's view.

194. D: Choices *B* and *D* are the most relevant to this statement. It's clear that the author believes that laws are imposed by people on people. There is no force or exterior presence giving laws power or upholding them. Law is the people's power and instrument alone. It's because of this that there is a fear element implied in the author's statement—the fear that there are consequences for going against this force that the people invented. This is the author's idea: that people give laws power, even though in reality, laws don't exist except for being made by man. The answer that best captures this is Choice *D*.

195. C: Again, one must be careful of falling into the trap of choosing an answer that doesn't fully or completely identify the author's motivation. Choice *A* is naturally a good choice—it's true, but perhaps there's a stronger answer. Always be wary of the easy answer, as this can be a trap. Choice *B* could hold truth, but this doesn't appear to be the primary reason for the author's writing. He's clearly writing for people who are at least somewhat familiar with *Paradise Lost*. Choice *B* is incorrect. Choice *D* is very compelling because this is an important factor for the interpretation of *Paradise Lost*. However, the author doesn't present this in a statement or actively pursue proving this idea. Merely, he states this as a cornerstone for interpreting the text and moves on to explore other interpretations. Choice *C* aptly sums up what the writer is doing in the passage.

196. B: This answer can be inferred simply by looking over the paragraph transitions the author employs. Rather than remain on specific authors for long stretches of time, the author provides a kind of snapshot of how people view Milton during certain periods of time. As discoveries are made, views change, and different trends begin, Milton's work is looked at differently. He doesn't go into detail with most of the writers, instead favoring to analyze shifts in Milton reception, which is key to the answer. Choice *B* is correct.

197. A: The conventional meaning of "mental constitution" refers to someone's mental wellness or even state of mind. However, this isn't the case here; plugging such terms into the sentence makes no sense.

To solve this riddle, one must look deeply into the context of what's being said. It's clear that the speaker isn't discussing mental states, but specific interests: "'Milton's mental constitution, then, demanded in the material upon which it was to work, a combination of qualities such as very few subjects could offer.'" Here the author directly states that only a few subjects really inspired his work. Thus, Choice *A* would be a promising alternative to "mental constitution."

198. D: Choice *D* is the most logical choice. Even if Milton didn't intend some moments of symbolism, this doesn't mean that the reader cannot identify with it. Literature to a degree is subjective by nature. If people can see symbolism in places where it might not have been intended, it can be inferred that they can prescribe multiple or alternative themes to the work as a whole in kind.

199. C: Again, the author doesn't so much take a stance on a particular view, so much as present several interpretations of themes and assess the levels in which they highlight the content of *Paradise Lost*. The author already admits that there are several interpretations of *Paradise Lost's* theme; therefore, it's conceivable that many "truths" can be drawn from the work, both literal and intended directly, unintentionally crafted through symbolism, or applied through metaphor. Therefore, Choice *C* is the most reasonable answer based on the passage content.

200. A: This kind of information would greatly explain how people interpret Milton and arrive at a theme or themes. Discussing Milton's specific style should be included in an area that focuses on the use or interpretation of artistic symbolism. Otherwise, this information would be out of place in the text. The best answer is Choice *A*. Recall that paragraph five discusses how *Paradise Lost* could be seen as "chiefly symbolic and poetic." A focus on style could expand upon this idea and add further clarification. Therefore, Choice *A* is the best answer.

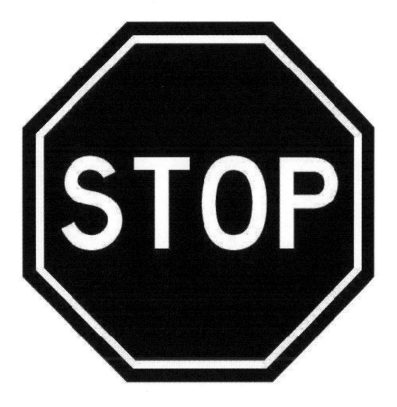

FREE Test Taking Tips DVD Offer

To help us better serve you, we have developed a Test Taking Tips DVD that we would like to give you for FREE. **This DVD covers world-class test taking tips that you can use to be even more successful when you are taking your test.**

All that we ask is that you email us your feedback about your study guide. Please let us know what you thought about it – whether that is good, bad or indifferent.

To get your **FREE Test Taking Tips DVD**, email freedvd@studyguideteam.com with "FREE DVD" in the subject line and the following information in the body of the email:

    a. The title of your study guide.

    b. Your product rating on a scale of 1-5, with 5 being the highest rating.

    c. Your feedback about the study guide. What did you think of it?

    d. Your full name and shipping address to send your free DVD.

If you have any questions or concerns, please don't hesitate to contact us at freedvd@studyguideteam.com.

Thanks again!